WITHDRAWN
UTSA LIBRARIES

P9-DTV-292

CLINICAL ASSESSMENT
AND MANAGEMENT OF
SEVERE PERSONALITY DISORDERS

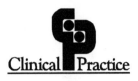

Clinical Practice

Number 35

Judith H. Gold, M.D., F.R.C.P.C.
Elissa P. Benedek, M.D.
Series Editors

CLINICAL ASSESSMENT
AND MANAGEMENT OF
SEVERE PERSONALITY DISORDERS

Edited by

Paul S. Links, M.D., M.Sc., F.R.C.P.C.

Washington, DC
London, England

Note: The authors have worked to ensure that all information in this book concerning drug dosages, schedules, and routes of administration is accurate as of the time of publication and consistent with standards set by the U.S. Food and Drug Administration and the general medical community. As medical research and practice advance, however, therapeutic standards may change. For this reason and because human and mechanical errors sometimes occur, we recommend that readers follow the advice of a physician who is directly involved in their care or the care of a member of their family.

Books published by the American Psychiatric Press, Inc., represent the views and opinions of the individual authors and do not necessarily represent the policies and opinions of the Press or the American Psychiatric Association.

Copyright © 1996 American Psychiatric Press, Inc.
ALL RIGHTS RESERVED
Manufactured in the United States of America on acid-free paper
First Edition   99 98 97 96   4 3 2 1

American Psychiatric Press, Inc.
1400 K Street, N.W., Washington, DC 20005

Library of Congress Cataloging-in-Publication Data
Clinical assessment and management of severe personality disorders /
 ˙ edited by Paul S. Links.
        p.   cm. — (Clinical practice series ; #35)
     Includes bibliographical references and index.
     ISBN 0-88048-488-8 (alk. paper)
     1. Personality disorders.   I. Links, Paul S.   II. Series:
Clinical practice ; no. 35
     [DNLM: 1. Personality Disorders—diagnosis.   2. Personality
Disorders—therapy.   W1 CL767J v.35 1996 / WM 190 C641 1996]
RC554.C56   1996
616.85′82—dc20
DNLM/DLC
for Library of Congress   95-19714
                                                                        CIP

British Library Cataloguing in Publication Data
A CIP record is available from the British Library.

Library
University of Texas
at San Antonio

Contents

Contributors

Stephen Allnutt, M.D., F.R.C.P.C.
Fellow, Forensic Psychiatry, Royal Ottawa Hospital, University of Ottawa, Ottawa, Ontario, Canada

Ingrid Boiago, B.A., R.N.
Clinical Research Nurse, Department of Psychiatry, McMaster University, Hamilton, Ontario, Canada

David Dawson, M.D., F.R.C.P.C.
Psychiatrist-in-Chief/Clinical Director, Hamilton Psychiatric Hospital; and Professor, Department of Psychiatry, McMaster University, Hamilton, Ontario, Canada

Paul S. Links, M.D., M.Sc., F.R.C.P.C.
Deputy Chief of Psychiatry, The Wellesley Hospital; and Professor, Department of Psychiatry, University of Toronto, Toronto, Ontario, Canada

M. Janice E. Mitton, B.A., R.N., M.H.Sc.
Clinical Research Nurse, Clinical Lecturer, Department of Psychiatry, McMaster University, Hamilton, Ontario, Canada

Jayne Patrick, Ph.D.
Staff Psychologist, Hamilton Psychiatric Hospital; and Associate Professor, Department of Psychiatry, McMaster University, Hamilton, Ontario, Canada

Kenneth R. Silk, M.D.
Chief, Adult Services; Director, Personality Disorders Program, University Medical Center; and Associate Professor, Department of Psychiatry, University of Michigan, Ann Arbor, Michigan

Robert van Reekum, M.D., F.R.C.P.C.
Staff Psychiatrist, Bay Crest Centre; and Assistant Professor, Department of Psychiatry, University of Toronto, Toronto, Ontario, Canada

Introduction
to the Clinical Practice Series

Over the years of its existence, the series of monographs entitled *Clinical Insights* has gradually become focused on providing current, factual, and theoretical material of interest to clinicians working outside of a hospital setting. To reflect this orientation, the name of the series has been changed to *Clinical Practice*.

The Clinical Practice Series will provide books that will give mental health clinicians a practical, clinical approach to a variety of psychiatric problems. These books will provide up-to-date literature reviews and emphasize the most recent treatment methods. Thus, the publications in the series should be of interest to clinicians working in both psychiatry and the other mental health professions.

Each year, a number of books in the series will be published on all aspects of clinical practice. In addition, from time to time when appropriate, these publications may be revised and updated. Thus, the series will provide quick access to relevant and important areas of psychiatric practice. Some books in the series will be authored by a person considered to be an expert in that particular area; others will be edited by such an expert, who will also draw together other knowledgeable authors to produce a comprehensive overview of that topic.

Some of the books in the Clinical Practice Series will have their foundation in presentations at an annual meeting of the American Psychiatric Association. All will contain the most recently available information on the subjects discussed. Theoretical and scientific data will be applied to clinical situations, and case illustrations will be utilized in order to make the material even more relevant for the practitioner. Thus, the Clinical Practice Series should provide educational reading in a compact format especially designed for the mental health clinician-psychiatrist.

Judith H. Gold, M.D., F.R.C.P.C.
Series Editor
Clinical Practice Series

Clinical Practice Series Titles

Clinical Assessment and Management of Severe Personality Disorders (#35)
Edited by Paul S. Links, M.D., M.Sc., F.R.C.P.C.

Predictors of Treatment Response in Mood Disorders (#34)
Edited by Paul J. Goodnick, M.D.

Successful Psychiatric Practice: Current Dilemmas, Choices, and Solutions (#33)
Edited by Edward K. Silberman, M.D.

Alternatives to the Hospital for Acute Psychiatric Treatment (#32)
Edited by Richard Warner, M.B., D.P.M.

Behavioral Complications in Alzheimer's Disease (#31)
Edited by Brian A. Lawlor, M.D.

Clinician Safety (#30)
Edited by Burr Eichelman, M.D., Ph.D.

Effective Use of Group Therapy in Managed Care (#29)
Edited by K. Roy MacKenzie, M.D., F.R.C.P.C.

Rediscovering Childhood Trauma: Historical Casebook and Clinical Applications (#28)
Edited by Jean M. Goodwin, M.D., M.P.H.

Treatment of Adult Survivors of Incest (#27)
Edited by Patricia L. Paddison, M.D.

Madness and Loss of Motherhood: Sexuality, Reproduction, and Long-Term Mental Illness (#26)
Edited by Roberta J. Apfel, M.D., M.P.H., and
Maryellen H. Handel, Ph.D.

Psychiatric Aspects of Symptom Management in Cancer Patients (#25)
Edited by William Breitbart, M.D., and Jimmie C. Holland, M.D.

Responding to Disaster: A Guide for Mental Health Professionals (#24)
Edited by Linda S. Austin, M.D.

Introduction

Paul S. Links, M.D., M.Sc., F.R.C.P.C.

*P*ersonality is the fulcrum on which our clinical work with patients balances. When patients do not respond to therapies, precipitate sleepless nights of worry, or cause clinicians to have an immediate reaction at the mention of the patient's name, we need to turn our attention to the personality attributes of the patient and how they affect our therapeutic work. Our own personality defines the equilibrium between our success and failures.

This book grew out of our need to respond to patients attending an outpatient clinic in a medium-sized urban setting. Our interest and respect for these patients came from observing their tireless efforts to be understood. Despite many failed attempts, these patients would rally for another try. We recognized the limits of our knowledge, and we sought a new way to respond to these patients.

Many of these patients had severe personality disorders. They had serious coexisting psychiatric problems, such as substance abuse or major psychiatric illnesses. Their histories indicated repeated hospitalizations, endless exposure to medications, and frequent evidence of self-destructive behaviors. These patients seldom held productive jobs, lived independently, or had supportive networks. Yet despite all these disadvantages, many maintained hope for a better future.

My colleagues and I turned to the existing literature but found little that was directed toward these patients. Most of the books theorized about intensive individual psychotherapy with patients who sounded much healthier than those we saw. We gained a better understanding but little practical help for planning for our next session. Our setting was not able to offer two to three sessions of psychotherapy per week. And our experience matched the little research evidence that was available: patients with severe personality disorders, such as borderline personality disorder, frequently dropped out of therapy within the first 6 months of treatment (Gunderson et al. 1989; Skodol et al. 1983), and 10% or fewer patients with severe personality disorders successfully completed psychotherapy (Waldinger and Gunderson 1984, 1987). We agreed that some patients benefited from intensive psychotherapy but that most did not.

My colleagues and I responded to the perceived gap in our knowledge by searching for new facts or theories to guide our work. Over the last 15 years, we have explored several research hypotheses related to borderline personality disorder. We are not alone in this venture. Blashfield (1993) documented the rapid growth rate of scientific literature on borderline personality disorder, which is doubling once every 8 years. Several professionals at McMaster University came together to develop a specialty assessment and consultation service, which we called the Personality Investigation Team (PIT), for patients with personality or behavior problems. For patients seen in our service, we tried to bring together the latest research and our growing clinical experience to meet the multitude of problems they experienced.

Many of my colleagues from this team have contributed to this volume. Much of what we learned we owe to our patients, who tolerated our endless questions and trusted us with their inner thoughts and feelings. Our colleague Dave Dawson conceptualized patients with personality disorders from a new perspective and developed a model of therapy called *relationship management.* His insights about the management of patients with borderline personality disorder are available in his recent publication (Dawson and MacMillan 1993). In this volume, Dr. Dawson has extended his relationship management model to assist clinicians in the management of patients with all types of severe personality disorders.

The overall objective of this book is to provide the clinician working in the community with clinical assessment and management approaches for patients with severe personality disorders.

Our goal was to provide a tool that would be of value for a variety of mental health clinicians, including psychiatrists, psychologists, social workers, nurse practitioners, and primary care physicians. We attempted to avoid psychiatric jargon and long, theoretical elaborations because we wanted the book to be of use for learners from the various disciplines. A few fundamental beliefs guide our work with these patients. These beliefs have been expressed by others and are principles of psychiatric rehabilitation (Links 1993) and the underpinnings of relationship management. However, these three fundamental beliefs cannot be overstated and are outlined as follows:

1. **Self-determination:** Patients with personality disorders should be active participants in all phases of treatment and rehabilitation. The patient should be treated as a competent adult. Encouraging this active involvement will reinforce the patient's feelings of empowerment and competence. Self-determination means that the patient should choose the areas to be targeted for treatment or rehabilitation. This approach helps the patient feel validated by others.
2. **Focus on role functioning:** Symptom status may be poorly related to the patient's functioning in the roles of daily life. Energies must be directed to understanding and assisting patients to improve their functioning. It may be important to help patients accept the symptoms and have realistic expectations about the value and purpose of interventions targeted at symptomatology.
3. **Maintaining hope:** Therapists often approach patients with personality disorders with a sense of hopelessness. Maintaining hope that the patient will get well is viewed by patients as a very helpful part of a constructive therapeutic relationship (Perry et al. 1990). Long-term follow-up studies have provided evidence that most borderline patients improve with time (Paris 1988). Therefore, for the individual patient, the therapist is justified in maintaining hope and the expectation that the patient may greatly improve.
   The therapist should maintain a longitudinal perspective of the patient's problems in order to maintain hope and accurately observe the patient's progress. There will often be oscillations in the patient-therapist relationship and in the

perceptions of progress. The therapist should retain a view of the patient's life course and understand that change may progress slowly and irregularly.

This book is organized into 10 chapters. The first five chapters focus on the clinical assessment of patients with suspected personality disorders. The final five chapters deal with issues related to the management of patients with severe personality disorders. In Chapter 1, Dr. Links and colleagues discuss the reasons for focusing on personality disorder diagnoses and discuss how the clinician can recognize a patient with a personality disorder from a clinical assessment. In Chapter 2, Drs. Allnutt and Links describe how a clinician can differentiate one personality disorder from another and make specific personality disorder diagnoses. The authors have suggested the use of the "optimal criterion" for this purpose. In Chapter 3, Dr. Patrick explains the use of psychological tests, both projective and empirically derived, to assist with the diagnosis and treatment of personality disorders. In Chapter 4, Dr. van Reekum introduces the neuropsychiatric perspective and how it relates to the assessment and management of patients with personality disorders. In Chapter 5, the frequent and complex clinical situation of managing a patient with both a symptom disorder and a personality disorder is examined. Dr. Silk, in Chapter 6, proposes an approach to the psychopharmacological management of patients with personality disorders. Chapters 7 and 8 address the management of patients with personality disorders in the community, in an inpatient setting, and most important, in the clinician's office. In these chapters, Dr. Dawson uses his model of relationship management to discuss how the clinician can work with patients with distressing personality disorders. In Chapter 9, Dr. Links and colleagues review the importance of a history of childhood sexual abuse and other childhood trauma. The etiological impact and the implications of this history for psychotherapeutic management are discussed. In Chapter 10, Ms. Mitton and Dr. Links discuss a framework for interacting and intervening with the families of patients with personality disorders.

I want to acknowledge the important contributions of my colleagues on the Personality Investigation Team and the Borderline Study Group, Department of Psychiatry, McMaster University, who have helped foster an interest and understanding of patients with personality disorders. I express my thanks to Mrs. Cyndi Gee, Mrs. Louise Woltman, and Mrs. Sheila Proctor for the many hours given to the preparation of this manuscript. Finally, I express my thanks to my family and the inspiration provided by my wife, Michelle; my two sons, Braedon and Duncan; and my new daughter, Madison, as I worked on editing this volume.

References

Blashfield R: Growth of the personality disorders literature from 1975 to 1991. Paper presented at the Third International Congress on the Disorders of Personality, Cambridge, MA, September 1993

Dawson DF, MacMillan HL: Relationship Management of the Borderline Patient: From Understanding to Treatment. New York, Brunner/Mazel, 1993

Gunderson JG, Frank AF, Ronningstam EF, et al: Early discontinuance of borderline patients from psychotherapy. J Nerv Ment Dis 177:38–42, 1989

Links PS: Psychiatric rehabilitation model for borderline personality disorder. Can J Psychiatry 38:S35–S38, 1993

Paris J: Follow-up studies of borderline personality disorder: a critical review. Journal of Personality Disorders 2:189–197, 1988

Perry JC, Herman JL, van der Kolk BA, et al: Psychotherapy and psychological trauma in borderline personality disorder. Psychiatric Annals 20:33–43, 1990

Skodol A, Buckley P, Charles E: Is there a characteristic pattern to the treatment history of clinical outpatients with borderline personality? J Nerv Ment Dis 171:405–410, 1983

Waldinger R, Gunderson JG: Completed psychotherapies with borderline patients. Am J Psychotherapy 38:190–202, 1984

Waldinger R, Gunderson JG: Successful Psychotherapy With Borderline Patients. New York, MacMillan, 1987

CHAPTER 1

Understanding and Recognizing Personality Disorders

Paul S. Links, M.D., M.Sc., F.R.C.P.C.
Ingrid Boiago, B.A., R.N.
Stephen Allnutt, M.D., F.R.C.P.C.

*P*ersonality disorders can be diagnosed in approximately 10%–15% of the general population (Reich et al. 1989; Weissman 1993). Within psychiatric services, most patients meet criteria for both a symptom disorder, such as major depression, and a personality disorder. Patients with personality disorders are often frequent service users; for example, Swartz et al. (1990) surveyed a community sample of adults and reported that respondents with borderline personality disorder had extremely high rates of mental health service usage, approaching those of respondents with schizophrenia. These patients not only are in great need of care but often are the most difficult and confusing for clinicians to treat. In order to better manage these patients, clinicians should understand the following:

- What is a personality disorder?
- Why is it important to recognize a patient with a personality disorder?

This chapter is a revision of the paper Links PS, Allnutt S: "Understanding Personality Disorders." *Medicine North America* 17:233–275, 1994, and is published with the permission of CME Publishing Ltd., Montreal, Quebec, Canada.

- How does a clinician recognize a patient with a personality disorder?

What Is a Personality Disorder?

Personality is the synthesis of our behaviors, cognitions, and emotions that makes each of us unique. These attributes tend to be stable and enduring, allowing our family, friends, and acquaintances to predict how we will respond to a given situation and permitting them to describe us to others.

Although our personalities allow others to predict and anticipate our responses to situations, a person with a "healthy" personality demonstrates a range of coping styles and a variety of responses when placed in stressful situations. A disorder of personality occurs when a person cannot display such flexibility and adaptability. The lack of adaptability and a limited repertoire of coping styles can result in distress for the individual or for those around him or her.

Personality disorders are generally recognizable by adolescence or earlier and continue throughout most of adulthood. They are deeply ingrained, inflexible, maladaptive patterns of sufficient severity to cause either impairment in functioning or profound distress.

Attempts at categorizing personality and developing typologies stretch back to Hippocrates' four temperaments. The nature of the typologies has varied from the four temperaments to Fourier's 810 character types. With a focus on abnormal behavior, the American Psychiatric Association developed a diagnostic classification system for personality disorders. The purpose was to assist clinicians in attending to this aspect of the patient's presentation and in separating personality features from symptom disorders. In 1980, DSM-III (American Psychiatric Association 1980) was developed. This classification system has been revised twice since 1980, with the publication of DSM-III-R (American Psychiatric Association 1987) and DSM-IV (American Psychiatric Association 1994a). With the publication of DSM-III, a separate diagnostic classification system was created for making personality disorder diagnoses (Axis II). Axis I in DSM-III was restricted to symptom disorder diagnoses, such as schizophrenia, mood disorders, and anxiety disorders. The creation of Axis II had the desired effect, and more clinical and research interest has been directed toward personality disorders.

The latest revision, DSM-IV, was completed in May 1994. In general, the classification of Axis II disorders has undergone only minor modifications as the DSM-IV Axis II Work Group aspired to a "conservative approach to change" (Gunderson and Shea 1991, p. 338). Modifications were made when empirical evidence supported the change and when the changes helped achieve the overall goal of increasing correspondence with the *International Classification of Diseases,* 10th Edition (ICD-10) (World Health Organization 1992), which was also under review (Gunderson and Shea 1991).

Clinicians who are already familiar with the terminology and categories of the earlier editions will have little difficulty using and comprehending the DSM-IV diagnoses. The *DSM-IV Update* (American Psychiatric Association 1994b) describes only three major changes to the DSM-III-R personality disorder diagnoses that were incorporated in DSM-IV. For antisocial personality disorder, the items "failure to sustain consistent work behavior or honor financial obligations" were collapsed into one item, and two items, "irresponsible parenting" and "failure to sustain a monogamous relationship," were deleted. One item covering transient, stress-related paranoid ideation or severe dissociative symptoms was added to the criteria for borderline personality disorder. The diagnosis of passive-aggressive personality disorder was deleted because the concept was believed to reflect a single personality trait rather than a cohesive disorder. The criteria for each of the disorders are given in Chapter 2.

The usefulness of personality disorder diagnoses for deciding on the management of patients is much in debate. Some authors have argued that the uniqueness of an individual's personality, both a person's strengths and weaknesses, are better captured with a dimensional approach (Widiger and Frances 1985). Although there are definite advantages to characterizing personality with a dimensional approach, we have argued for retaining diagnoses to assist clinical decision making (Gunderson et al. 1991). Many of the decisions facing a clinician are "yes/no" decisions—for example, deciding whether medication should be prescribed or hospitalization arranged. For these decisions, the determination of the diagnosis will be of use to the clinician. The reader will note that the book presents our ideas about management with a medical diagnostic approach.

Why Is It Important to Recognize a Patient With a Personality Disorder?

The diagnosis of a personality disorder may indicate that the patient is at increased risk for completed suicide, affect the course and response to treatment of coexisting disorders, highlight important etiological factors, inform the clinician about the patient's course and outcome, indicate areas of significant social role dysfunction, and assist with the clinician's overall management of the patient.

Risk of Completed Suicide

Certain personality disorders place patients at chronic risk for suicidal behaviors. Patients with borderline personality disorder frequently exhibit suicidal or self-destructive behaviors, and approximately 10% of patients with borderline personality disorder will successfully complete suicide over the course of their illness (Paris 1988).

The acute suicidal risk in a patient with chronic suicidal behaviors needs to be carefully assessed. The importance of the suicidal behavior is sometimes underestimated or dismissed during the emergency room assessment if the patient is suspected of having antisocial and/or borderline personality disorder. The particularly high risk for completed suicide faced by these patients makes this a potentially dangerous attitude. The presence of a personality disorder is, in fact, likely to increase the risk that the patient may go on to complete suicide.

Careful attention must be given to the situation and circumstances around the current suicide threat or attempt. Information must be obtained about the patient's previous suicide attempts and their magnitude of lethality. A patient's suicidal behaviors often follow a very repetitive pattern. Some patients with severe personality disorders make repeated suicidal attempts that are of high lethality. One patient in particular periodically acted on her chronic suicidal thoughts. She usually did this within the context of her therapist's summer vacation. On one occasion, she sent via facsimile transmission a vague threat of suicide to her lawyer, who then proceeded to contact her vacationing therapist. Although the communication ended up being a cry for help and was directly related to the therapist's absence, her risk for completed suicide was very real. In the past, the patient had taken enormous quantities of medication and would make a call for help just before succumbing to the medication. As this example demonstrates, one needs to assess the circumstances and lethality of previous attempts in order to respond to the current situation.

Patients often present suicidal behaviors when they are trying to effect changes in their environment. They use their threats or behaviors in an attempt to maintain a relationship and deal with their fear of being rejected (Gunderson 1984). These suicidal behaviors have a manipulative quality, and often strategies can be developed to help the patient effect changes in a more constructive way. The risk of completed suicide is usually lower when the behavior is an attempt to manipulate the environment. The risk of completed suicide appears to be heightened when the patient perceives that he or she has, or when he or she in fact has, suffered a major loss. The patient's experience of a major loss can be very disorganizing and can precipitate psychotic phenomena. Under these circumstances, the patient can be more self-destructive and less responsive to any environmental change. If the patient is considered to be responding to perceived or real losses, interventions may be required to ensure his or her safety.

Some factors appear to increase the risk of suicide in certain patients with severe personality disorders. A patient with borderline personality disorder complicated by a major depression is at increased risk for suicidal behaviors or even completed suicide; in such a patient, persistent reports of depression accompanied by suicidal thoughts signal a particularly high risk. The drug and alcohol abuse that often accompanies these personality disorders further increases the risk of suicide (Stone 1990). There is some evidence that the risk of completed suicide in this patient group increases around the time of hospitalizations and shortly after discharge.

The chronic risk of suicide can be more of an issue for the clinician than for the patient. For many patients with severe personality disorders who persistently contemplate suicide, these thoughts are a coping strategy that gives them a sense of power and control over their life experiences (Paris 1993). They often struggle against the clinician's attempts to control or modify these thoughts. The clinician must monitor this risk faced by the patient over time. The clinician's other important task, however, is to understand what these chronic suicidal thoughts mean to the patient. Therapeutic gains are possible as a patient comes to understand the meaning behind these thoughts.

Coexisting Disorders

The coexistence of a symptom disorder and a personality disorder will have important implications for the treatment and course of the symptom disorder. There is considerable evidence that the co-occurrence of a symptom disorder (e.g., major depression) with a personality disorder lessens the response to standard therapies, delays the response to treatment, and increases the risk of recurrence of the symptom disorder (see Chapter 5 for a further discussion of comorbidity). These effects on treatment response and course of the symptom disorder seem to occur regardless of the precise nature of either the symptom disorder or the coexisting personality disorder (Reich and Green 1991). It may be important to impart such information to the patient; for example, the patient should know that antidepressant medication, although likely to reduce the symptoms of depression, will often not alleviate them completely. Most patients should anticipate trying the medication for 4–6 weeks before expecting any changes to occur.

Etiology of Personality Disorders

Understanding the etiology of personality disorders is one of the most challenging areas of inquiry for both researchers and clinicians. Etiological models must go beyond linear cause-and-effect relations to integrate an array of biopsychosocial factors. Several general principles, however, can guide our development of etiological models.

First, a substantial genetic basis of personality has been shown for normal personality traits; based on studies of healthy twins, heritabilities for traits range from 40% to 60% (Plomin 1990). Livesley et al. (1993) reported similar results for 12 of 18 dimensions of personality disorders, with heritabilities ranging from 40% to 60%. The influence of genetic factors varied widely across traits; callousness had an additive genetic effect of 56%, whereas that of conduct problems was 0%.

Second, the developmental impact of the child's family environment is an important etiological factor in the genesis of severe personality disorders. The etiological models, however, must move beyond a focus on a specific phase of development; for example, the separation-individuation phase. Rather, they must integrate the host of risk factors and/or traumatic events that interact and lead to psychopathology (Links and Munroe-Blum 1990; Links and van Reekum 1993). Livesley et al. (1993) found that nonshared environmental influences, such as differential parental care between twins, for the different dimensions of personality pathology ranged from 36% to 71%. The neurodevelopmental factors in the etiology of personality disorders are discussed in Chapter 4. The possible role of childhood sexual abuse in the etiology of borderline personality disorder is discussed in detail in Chapter 9.

Third, broader social factors, such as rapid social change that interferes with intergenerational transmission of values (Millon 1987), must be integrated into the etiological models. Paris (1992) indicated that social factors are not independent causal determinants, but they lower thresholds for other risk factors to act on the development of psychopathology.

Fourth, those factors that determine the course of psychopathology are likely to be separate and distinct from etiological factors. In addition to being biopsychosocial factors that impinge on the course of personality disorders, these factors may change over time. For example, early in the course of borderline personality disorder, high levels of impulsivity may be predictive of poor outcome. By the fourth decade, however, as the impulsive aspects "burn out," the affective psychopathology may become more predictive of the long-term course (Links et al. 1993).

Two current models of personality disorder are worthy of mention because of their integration of biopsychosocial factors. Cloninger (1987) developed a "unified biosocial theory of personality" based on three underlying genetic dimensions of personality called "novelty seeking, harm avoidance, and reward dependence" (p. 574). Besides being based on the pattern of response to conditioned signals of punishment, reward, and novelty, the three dimensions were hypothesized to be related to separate monoamine neuromodulator systems: novelty seeking was suggested to relate to the dopamine system; harm avoidance, to the serotonin system; and reward dependence, to the norepinephrine system. Siever and Davis (1991) developed an integrated model of personality disorders based on the proposition that "personality disorders can be formulated as a dimensional model grounded in the major Axis I syndromes" (p. 1648). The dimensions were conceptualized as a continuum, with Axis I disorders on the extreme end of the continuum and milder, persistent disorders, characterized as Axis II disorders, at the other end of the continuum. The four dimensions making up the core psychobiological predispositions were 1) cognitive/perceptual organization, 2) affective instability, 3) impulsivity/aggression, and 4) anxiety/inhibition. Each of the dimensions is related to particular Axis I and II disorders, biological indexes, and characteristic coping strategies (Siever and Davis 1991). As with Siever's model, future etiological models of personality disorder must explain the relation between Axis I and II disorders, and a single model may not be sufficient to explain these relations (see Chapter 5 for a further discussion of comorbidity).

Course and Outcome

By definition, personality disorders are said to begin by late adolescence and continue throughout much of adulthood. The course and outcome of the more severe personality disorders, however, have been clarified by recent research (Stone 1993). Many of the personality disorders are not as chronic and unremitting as was first thought. Sharing this information can maintain the patient's and the clinician's hopes for change. Being informed about the course of the disorder, the clinician will be able to anticipate the patient's rate of change over time.

The course of borderline personality disorder has been carefully studied. Borderline personality disorder usually begins in late adolescence or early adulthood, and the initial course is typically stormy and crisis ridden. Most patients, if they require hospitalization during this period, will continue to have markedly impaired functioning for the first 2 years after their hospitalization (Links et al. 1990). Patients with initially high levels of impulsivity or a history of outpatient psychiatric contact in childhood were found to be at greater risk for continuation of borderline psychopathology over the early course of their disorder (Links et al. 1993). The risk of completed suicide appears to be higher during the first 5–7 years of the disorder (Stone 1990). Over longer periods of follow-up, however, borderline patients seem to do surprisingly well. Summarizing the four major follow-up studies, Paris (1988) indicated that approximately half of patients with an initial diagnosis of borderline personality disorder will be functioning normally by their fourth decade of life. Although most patients do well, approximately one-third with borderline personality disorder will still show significant role dysfunction and considerable psychopathology on follow-up. It is unclear at present why some patients with borderline personality disorder improve over time and others do not.

The course of antisocial personality disorder has been characterized as "burning out" in midlife (Robins 1966). Although these patients may demonstrate less antisocial behavior by midlife, they remain severely impaired. Black et al. (1993) followed up patients with antisocial personality disorder some 30 years after their initial assessment. On follow-up, these individuals showed marked areas of social dysfunction and relationship difficulties.

Stone (1993) reviewed the long-term outcomes of patients with personality disorders and concluded that little is known about the course and outcome of patients with less severe personality disorders, particularly those who receive only outpatient care. Schizotypal personality disorder appears to run a chronic course, and McGlashan (1986) found the outcomes for these patients to be only slightly better than those for patients with schizophrenia. Wolff and Chick (1980) followed patients with schizoid personality disorder from childhood to adulthood and found these personality traits to be very stable over time. Plakun (1989) reported that patients with narcissistic personality disorder had higher rates of readmission over a 15-year follow-up period than did patients with borderline personality disorder. Narcissistic patients reported poorer functioning and less sexual satisfaction than did borderline patients on follow-up.

Social Role Dysfunction

By definition, the diagnosis of personality disorders should lead to distress or impairment in social functioning. Very little is known, however, about the relation between diagnoses of personality disorder and performance in social roles, perhaps with the exception of borderline personality disorder. Results of previous long-term follow-up studies have suggested that borderline patients are less dysfunctional in work roles than in social, leisure, and family roles (McGlashan 1985; Paris et al. 1987; Stone 1990). Stone (1990), however, characterized the work functioning of the borderline patients from his follow-up study by concluding that "many of the patients at follow-up were accomplishing in their 30s what their high-school classmates were able to complete in their 20s" (p. 32). The status of symptoms, particularly of affective and impulsive symptoms, was highly correlated with role performance in our sample of patients with borderline personality disorder, who were assessed 2 years after discharge from an inpatient service (Links 1993).

Role performance may also be context bound; for example, a patient with paranoid personality disorder may generally be isolated and friendless but make an excellent night watchman, enjoying the solitude but also accepting the need for vigilance through the long night hours. The clinician should pay attention to the patient's role functioning. Patients should be asked about their functioning in each of their roles, including family life, intimate relationships, work, social/leisure, and financial functioning. By informing ourselves about where the patient has difficulty functioning, we can target the interventions at these areas.

Appropriate Management

The diagnosis of a personality disorder should help the clinician formulate an appropriate management plan for the patient. Much has been written about the management of borderline personality disorder. Blashfield (1993) found that literature on borderline personality disorder has had the fastest growth rate of all the literature on personality disorders and is doubling once every 8 years. Therefore, this diagnosis can be very informative. Patients with borderline personality disorder are liable to develop crises, seek hospitalization, and regress while on an inpatient unit. These patients stimulate strong countertransference reactions from the clinician, who should be alert for this eventuality. These patients often pressure clinicians to modify and violate clinician-patient boundaries. The clinician may need to be extra vigilant in practicing risk management strategies. The following vignette illustrates this point.

Case 1

Ms. A, a 39-year-old single mother, was sent to our consultation service for diagnostic assessment. In fact, her current therapist had labeled her as having borderline personality disorder after her "fit of rage" during a recent therapy session. This session led to the therapist's request for diagnostic clarification.

Ms. A presented with an array of symptoms and behavioral problems. She experienced dramatic mood swings. She frequently contemplated suicide, abused pain medication, and mutilated herself but took great care to conceal her wounds. Ms. A often failed to meet her responsibilities in her work or at home.

Ms. A had been physically abused as a child but denied any recollections of sexual abuse. Her history was a constant repetition of self-damaging relationships. She married at a young age to escape the tyranny at home, but her first two relationships were with physically abusive men. Ms. A was victimized by a minister who beseeched her to become sexually involved with him and with other parishioners. She reported being sexually abused by a professor while she was attending a university. Although she had seen a handful of therapists, she had recently ended an 8-year therapy relationship. From the history, this therapy coincided with a very stable, productive period in her life. Ms. A had abruptly ended the therapy relationship when she had been offered "more intensive" therapy by a counselor who had completed a short course of therapy with Ms. A's daughter. Ms. A's understanding that a promise had been made for more intensive work and more frequent sessions became increasingly demanding of the counselor.

Given the recurrent pattern of boundary violations perpetrated against this patient, we took great care to clarify our role and Ms. A's expectations of the consultation. We endeavored to have two team members present at each meeting to ensure that our communications were clear and consistent. The diagnosis of borderline personality disorder was confirmed. We encouraged the patient to reexamine her current needs for therapy and the benefits she received from the 8-year therapy with a therapist who appeared to manage the boundaries in the patient-therapist relationship.

The chapters that follow deal with other aspects of the management of patients with severe personality disorders. This book reflects the current state of knowledge about personality disorders, much of which pertains to patients with borderline personality disorder. The discussion of management approaches, however, addresses the management of a range of patients with severe personality disorders.

How Does the Clinician Recognize a Patient With a Personality Disorder?

Diagnosing a personality disorder from a clinical interview is difficult. The clinician may know the patient only from periodic office visits and see the patient only when he or she is having difficulty coping. The clinician should answer the following three questions when trying to assess a patient for a personality disorder:

1. Is a symptom disorder present?
2. Why is the patient seeking help?
3. How does the patient make me feel?

Is a Symptom Disorder Present?

Symptom disorders, such as major depression, often coexist with diagnoses of personality disorders, and the traits of each may overlap considerably. For example, a manic patient may be angry and impulsive, just as a patient with borderline personality disorder may be angry and impulsive.

Specific information about the onset and progression of symptoms, the repetitiveness and duration of the clinical picture, and the way in which symptoms relate to the patient's environment will help the clinician differentiate between a symptom disorder and the traits of a personality disorder. Symptom disorders are generally of recent onset and can be assessed by taking the history of present illness and examining the mental status. The traits of a personality disorder will have been evident for at least 3–5 years and are uncovered during the developmental, personal, and social history. Careful attention should be paid to the patient's pattern of relating to, perceiving, and thinking about his or her significant relationships. The personality disorder traits will wax and wane over a matter of days, but historically these traits will have surfaced repeatedly since early adulthood.

The distinction between a symptom disorder and the traits of a personality disorder can be difficult to make, and often the symptoms of a disorder are mistakenly attributed to a personality disorder. The two case vignettes that follow illustrate this point.

Case 2

Ms. B, a 28-year-old woman, reported that her main problem was her "moods." Usually she saw herself as sociable, functioning well, interested in activities, and although not happy, at least content. Ms. B reported chronic feelings of low self-esteem and shyness but felt she was usually able to cope well.

Then gradually, and usually with no identifiable precipitant, she noticed changes in her behavior and mood. She stopped eating properly, consuming either too much or too little, and her sleep became disrupted. Her behavior became uncharacteristic in that she stopped paying bills, let the house become dirty, and missed days at work. After these changes, she began to think negatively about other people and herself. She was unable to cope, cried easily, and could not make decisions. When these changes become unbearable, she tried to hurt herself by cutting her skin with a razor or to kill herself by taking a drug overdose or jumping in front of a car. She developed persistent thoughts that her insides were rotting. These changes in mood and behavior lasted a few weeks to months.

During these episodes, Ms. B became very demanding and dependent on her therapist and her boyfriend. She had interpersonal relationship problems related to work and impulsively quit jobs on occasion. She tended to abuse alcohol with this change in her mood.

Psychological testing reports were extremely positive for borderline personality disorder. Ms. B reported unstable and intense interpersonal relationships, impulsiveness, affective instability, intense anger, marked identity disturbance, and frantic efforts to avoid real or imagined abandonment.

Others believed Ms. B's behavior was becoming more problematic and frequent, but Ms. B thought that her depression was most significant. After a course of antidepressant therapy, when she no longer showed evidence of major depression, Ms. B no longer met the criteria for borderline personality disorder.

The diagnosis of personality disorder is more often made clinically and from psychological testing if the patient is assessed during a major depression. The depression creates a negative view of self and others and dramatically impairs interpersonal functioning. The preceding vignette highlights the importance of separating the current presentation from a longitudinal view of the patient's coping. Because of the difficulty separating the symptom disorder from a personality disorder, however, the clinician is often wise to forego diagnosing a personality disorder until after the patient has recovered from the depressive episode.

Case 3

Ms. C, an 18-year-old female inpatient, was referred to the Personality Investigation Team for assessment of her borderline personality disorder. Her admission followed her second overdose in the past year. A year before her admission, she had disclosed an incestuous relationship with her 16-year-old brother. Adding to the trauma, Ms. C reported that, of the family of nine, she had been close only to this brother. The familial conflict that followed the revelation of the abuse estranged her from her brother and forced her to move from the family home to live with friends.

Ms. C had functioned without difficulty until the past year. Now she complained of irritability, angry outbursts, dysphoric mood, guilt over her relationship with her brother, self-loathing, sleep disturbance, weight loss after loss of appetite, and increasing suicidal ideation. She also began to cut her arms.

The admission diagnosis was borderline personality disorder with dysthymia. During the 3-month stay on the ward, Ms. C was withdrawn, irritable, and quick to anger and attempted to overdose twice more, on both occasions calmly informing staff about the overdose directly after ingesting the pills. The patient received no medication and was discharged without follow-up, with a diagnosis of borderline personality disorder.

The preceding case illustrates the diagnostic dilemma confronting the clinician. Although a history of incest and sexual abuse is often found in patients with borderline personality disorder, this patient showed no evidence of this disorder before her crisis, a year before her admission. Individuals respond to crises in varying ways, and not always adaptively. Although this does not necessarily mean that their response is evidence of a personality disorder, it may reflect the state of the person during a life crisis.

The index behavior must have been present for at least 3–5 years to be regarded as a personality trait. Borderline traits in adolescent patients have been shown to be very changeable over time and may not indicate the beginnings of a stable and enduring personality disorder (Mattanah et al. 1995). Ms. C developed a major depression and expressed her subjective experience in a maladaptive way. The short duration of these behaviors suggested a symptom disorder rather than traits of a personality disorder. In such a case, a diagnosis of borderline personality disorder should be withheld and the patient reassessed after the depression has resolved.

The patient's self-abusive acts, suicidal behavior, withdrawal from staff, irritability, and affective instability made her a difficult patient. Patients who are difficult can trigger, in even the most experienced clinicians, feelings of resentment, frustration, or helplessness that can prompt a hastily arrived-at label of borderline personality disorder. Not all difficult patients are borderline, and not all borderline patients are difficult. To avoid this pitfall, the clinician should carefully document that the patient meets the DSM-IV criteria for borderline personality disorder.

The presentation of a patient with a personality disorder may depend on the context in which the patient is assessed. The patient with a personality disorder may appear impaired in one context but may function completely normally in another. A symptom disorder, however, will be independent of the context and will run a course of several weeks or months. The patient should be assessed several times over 2–3 weeks to help differentiate a symptom disorder from a personality disorder.

Why Is the Patient Seeking Help?

The clinician must understand the reasons that the patient is seeking help. The patient may be distressed and requesting help to end his or her distress. In such situations, the patient's symptoms are said to be *egodystonic*. This presentation is more characteristic of the anxious cluster of personality disorders, such as avoidant and obsessive-compulsive personality disorders. Other patients present for help because of the distress they cause to others rather than to themselves. These patients' symptoms or behaviors are characterized as being *egosyntonic*. These individuals are likely to have been encouraged by others to seek help and often do so only to protect themselves from retribution. Patients with personality disorders from the so-called dramatic cluster, such as antisocial or borderline personality disorders, are more likely to present in this way.

How Does the Patient Make Me Feel?

The assessment of the patient begins the moment he or she enters the room. The clinician's initial impressions of a patient's demeanor, dress, and behavior can provide clues to help understand the person's personality traits. Is the patient slow to make eye contact? How does he or she respond to cues such as initial greetings, questions, nods, and smiles? Is the patient overly familiar with the interviewer? Is the patient suspicious, withdrawn, and timid?

Clinicians can learn a great deal by monitoring their own responses to patients. It is not uncommon for a clinician to feel as though the patient is coercing him or her into acting in a certain way during interactions. For example, the clinician may feel pressured to take more and more control if the patient presents himself or herself as extremely helpless. Attempts by the clinician to help the patient are often ineffective in resolving the patient's helplessness and leave the clinician frustrated and angry. At its worst, this type of interaction can lead the clinician to transgress professional boundaries—for example, by trying to settle the patient with a soothing caress or by becoming angry and acting unprofessionally.

Patients who coerce the clinician into taking charge but then frustrate the clinician's attempts to do so are defending themselves from the very same feelings that such interactions evoke in the clinician. Rather than acknowledge feeling out of control, frustrated, or angry, the patient coerces someone else into experiencing these feelings. This is achieved by behaving in a manner that pressures other people to respond. The clinician's frustration and anger at his or her failed efforts accentuates the patient's attempts to fight off acknowledging these feelings within himself or herself.

By looking at where this type of interaction comes from, the clinician can use it to better understand the patient. The clinician who recognizes this pattern of interaction can try to label the patient's feelings, although the patient will often deny their existence. Acknowledgment by the clinician that he or she feels pressured to respond in a certain way will often free the patient to discuss his or her own feelings. This type of interaction, although difficult, can clarify a possible diagnosis; for example, clinicians will often be made to feel coerced by patients with borderline personality disorder. Through this interaction, the clinician may become more in touch with the patient's inner feeling state and self-experience.

Conclusion

If clinicians have an understanding of what their patients with personality disorders are experiencing, they will have a better chance of assisting these patients. Understanding what a personality disorder is, what the implications of this diagnosis are, and how to recognize a personality disorder will assist clinicians in their work with such patients. In Chapter 2, the authors address how clinicians can diagnose specific personality disorders and differentiate one diagnosis from another.

References

American Psychiatric Association: Diagnostic and Statistical Manual of Mental Disorders, 3rd Edition. Washington, DC, American Psychiatric Association, 1980

American Psychiatric Association: Diagnostic and Statistical Manual of Mental Disorders, 3rd Edition, Revised. Washington, DC, American Psychiatric Association, 1987

American Psychiatric Association: Diagnostic and Statistical Manual of Mental Disorders, 4th Edition. Washington, DC, American Psychiatric Association, 1994a

American Psychiatric Association: DSM-IV Update: Task Force on the Diagnostic and Statistical Manual of Mental Disorders, Fourth Edition. Washington, DC, American Psychiatric Press, 1994b

Black DW, Baumgard C, Bell SE: A follow-up study of antisocial personality disorder. Paper presented at the 146th annual meeting of the American Psychiatric Association, San Francisco, CA, May 1993

Blashfield R: Growth of the personality disorders literature from 1975 to 1991. Paper presented at the Third International Congress on the Disorder of Personality, Cambridge, MA, September 1993

Cloninger CR: A systematic method for clinical description and classification of personality variants. Arch Gen Psychiatry 44:573–588, 1987

Gunderson JG: Borderline Personality Disorder. Washington, DC, American Psychiatric Press, 1984

Gunderson JG, Shea MT: DSM-IV reviews of the personality disorders: introduction to the second part of the special series. Journal of Personality Disorders 5:337–339, 1991

Gunderson JG, Links PS, Reich JH: Competing models of personality disorders. Journal of Personality Disorders 5:60–68, 1991

Links PS: Psychiatric rehabilitation model for borderline personality disorder. Can J Psychiatry 38:S35–S38, 1993

Links PS, Munroe-Blum H: Family environment and borderline personality disorder: development of etiologic models, in Family Environment and Borderline Personality Disorder. Edited by Links PS. Washington, DC, American Psychiatric Press, 1990, pp 1–24

Links PS, van Reekum R: Childhood sexual abuse, parental impairment and the development of borderline personality disorder. Can J Psychiatry 38:472–474, 1993

Links PS, Mitton JE, Steiner M: Predicting outcome for borderline personality. Compr Psychiatry 31:490–498, 1990

Links PS, Mitton MJE, Steiner M: Stability of borderline personality disorder. Can J Psychiatry 38:255–259, 1993

Livesley WJ, Jang KL, Jackson DN, et al: Genetic and environmental contributions to dimensions of personality disorder. Am J Psychiatry 150:1826–1831, 1993

Mattanah JJF, Becker DF, Levy KN, et al: Diagnostic stability in adolescents followed up 2 years after hospitalization. Am J Psychiatry 152:889–894, 1995

McGlashan TH (ed): The prediction of outcome in borderline personality disorder: part V of the Chestnut Lodge follow-up study, in The Borderline: Current Empirical Research. Washington, DC, American Psychiatric Press, 1985, pp 61–98

McGlashan TH: Chestnut Lodge followup study, VI: long-term follow-up perspectives. Arch Gen Psychiatry 43:329–334, 1986

Millon T: On the genesis and prevalence of borderline personality disorder: a social learning thesis. Journal of Personality Disorders 1:354–372, 1987

Paris J: Follow-up studies of borderline personality disorder: a critical review. Journal of Personality Disorders 2:189–197, 1988

Paris J: Social risk factors for borderline personality disorder: a review and hypothesis. Can J Psychiatry 37:510–515, 1992

Paris J: Management of acute and chronic suicidality in patients with borderline personality disorder, in Borderline Personality Disorder: Etiology and Treatment. Edited by Paris J. Washington, DC, American Psychiatric Press, 1993, pp 373–384

Paris J, Brown R, Nowlis D: Long-term follow-up of borderline patients in a general hospital. Compr Psychiatry 28:530–535, 1987

Plakun EM: Narcissistic personality disorder: a validity study and comparison to borderline personality disorder. Psychiatr Clin North Am 12:603–620, 1989

Plomin R: The role of inheritance in behavior. Science 248:183–188, 1990

Reich JH, Green AI: Effect of personality disorders on outcome of treatment. J Nerv Ment Dis 179:74–82, 1991

Reich J, Yates W, Nduagube M: Prevalence of DSM-III personality disorders in the community. Soc Psychiatry Psychiatr Epidemiol 24:12–16, 1989

Robins LN: Deviant Children Grown Up. Baltimore, MD, Williams & Wilkins, 1966

Siever LS, Davis KL: A psychobiologic perspective on the personality disorders. Am J Psychiatry 148:1647–1658, 1991

Stone MH: The Fate of Borderline Patients. New York, Guilford, 1990

Stone MH: The long-term outcome in personality disorders. Br J Psychiatry 162:299–313, 1993

Swartz M, Blazer D, George L, et al: Estimating the prevalence of borderline personality disorder in the community. Journal of Personality Disorders 4:257–272, 1990

Weissman MM: The epidemiology of personality disorders: a 1990 update. Journal of Personality Disorders 7 (suppl):44–62, 1993

Widiger T, Frances A: The DSM-III personality disorders: perspectives from psychology. Arch Gen Psychiatry 42:615–623, 1985

Wolff S, Chick J: Schizoid personality in childhood: a controlled follow-up study. Psychol Med 10:85–100, 1980

World Health Organization: The ICD-10 Classification of Mental and Behavioural Disorders. Geneva, World Health Organization, 1992

CHAPTER 2

Diagnosing Specific Personality Disorders and the Optimal Criteria

Stephen Allnutt, M.D., F.R.C.P.C.
Paul S. Links, M.D., M.Sc., F.R.C.P.C.

Chapter 1 served to raise the clinician's index of suspicion that a patient has a personality disorder. The next step in the assessment of a patient is to diagnose the specific personality disorder that explains the patient's distress or dysfunction.

Pigeonholing patients into categories of particular personality disorders is challenging for the clinician to do on the basis of one or even several clinical encounters. Often personality difficulties are very context bound, and a patient with a personality disorder appears very different from one situation to another. Most patients with severe personality disorders meet the criteria for two or more personality disorder diagnoses (Perry 1990). The clinician must have some way of determining which personality disorder diagnosis should be the focus of concern.

It would be impossible for the clinician to keep track of the diagnostic criteria that need to be assessed to apply specific diagnoses. DSM-IV (American Psychiatric Association 1994) has 10 separate categories and more than 100 criteria in total to be

We gratefully acknowledge data provided by Dr. Bruce Pfohl on the prototypicality and positive predictive value of diagnostic criteria derived from research with the Structured Interview for Diagnosing Personality—Revised.

assessed. Many of the criteria are complex and require considerable clinical inference to establish their presence. Although improvements have been made since DSM-III (American Psychiatric Association 1980), many of the disorders are conceptually closely allied, and some criteria seem to overlap with one another. For example, the social discomfort of a patient with schizotypal personality disorder who has paranoid fears must be differentiated from the fear of embarrassment of a patient with avoidant personality disorder.

How, then, can the clinician come to differentiate one personality disorder from another? Three steps are suggested to assist the clinician in recognizing specific personality disorders during the clinical interview.

1.   Be aware of the factors that raise the suspicion of the presence of one personality disorder over another.
2.   Use the optimal criterion during the clinical interview.
3.   After the clinical interview, apply the full DSM-IV criteria for the specific personality disorder to confirm the diagnosis.

Before we review the steps, we need to explain what we mean by the term *optimal criterion*. Diagnosing personality disorders would be easier if the clinician had to remember only one criterion for each personality disorder. The clinician could then test for the presence or absence of the criterion and quickly diagnose the personality disorder. However, personality disorders are diagnosed by the presence of a collection of traits and not by a single criterion. It might be possible, however, to determine the one criterion for each personality disorder that would be most useful to remember as an aid to diagnosis. This one criterion, if found to be present from the clinical interview, would increase the probability that the personality disorder diagnosis exists. Such a criterion could be termed the optimal criterion (Table 2–1).

The prototypical model of classification used for personality disorders in DSM-IV means that not all criteria are required to make the diagnosis and that patients receiving the same diagnosis will meet different criteria for the disorder. Therefore, patients with the same diagnosis are very heterogeneous. In the classical model of classification, diagnoses are homogeneous, all patients have the same defining features, and all characteristics must be

Table 2–1. Optimal criteria for DSM-IV personality disorders

Personality disorder	Optimal criterion
Antisocial	Criminal, aggressive, impulsive, irresponsible behaviors
Avoidant	Avoids occupational activities that involve significant interpersonal contact because of fear of criticism, disapproval, or rejection
Borderline	Frantic efforts to avoid real or imagined abandonment
Dependent	Needs others to assume responsibility for most major areas of his or her life
Histrionic	Is uncomfortable in situations in which he or she is not the center of attention
Narcissistic	Has a grandiose sense of self-importance
Obsessive-compulsive	Shows perfectionism that interferes with task completion
Paranoid	Suspects, without sufficient basis, that others are exploiting, harming, or deceiving him or her
Schizoid	Neither desires nor enjoys close relationships, including being part of a family
Schizotypal	Odd thinking and speech: behavior or appearance that is odd, eccentric, or peculiar

present to make the diagnosis. Widiger and Frances (1985) suggested that the criteria used in a prototypical model should have certain characteristics to be diagnostically useful. Extending these characteristics, we have selected one criterion from each personality disorder that is the optimal criterion to remember and utilize in the clinical interview.

The optimal criterion was chosen for the following characteristics:

- *Prototypical*—Widiger and Frances (1985) consider a criterion as prototypical if the item has a relatively high correlation with the sum of all the criteria in the diagnosis and a relatively low correlation with the criteria for other personality disorder diagnoses. For the purposes of defining optimal criteria to use in the clinical interview, we chose a criterion that was believed to be conceptually related to the other criteria for that diagnosis. For example, the presence of the optimal criterion would help the clinician anticipate some of the other diagnostic features that should be considered to establish the specific diagnosis.
- *Behavioral description*—A criterion that describes specific behaviors is more objective, offers the best interrater reliability, and requires less inference.
- *High positive predictive value*—The positive predictive value (PPV) is the probability that patients who are positive for the particular criterion will have the target diagnosis. In other words, it indicates the degree of usefulness of the criterion in identifying those individuals who genuinely have the condition. A high PPV implies a low rate of false-negative results (i.e., those who actually have the target diagnosis but are found to be negative for this criterion) and a high rate of true-positive results (i.e., those who have the target diagnosis and are found to be positive for the criterion).

In deciding on the optimal criterion for each personality disorder diagnosis, we chose the criterion based on its prototypicality, examined data on the criterion's PPV, and favored behaviorally oriented characteristics. Data on the prototypicality and PPV of diagnostic criteria were derived from research with the Structured Interview for Diagnosing Personality—Revised (an instrument based on DSM-III-R [American Psychiatric Association 1987] diagnoses).

As mentioned, PPV is the probability that the test will be positive (i.e., that the criterion will be present) if the patient has the index diagnosis. It must be borne in mind, however, that the diagnostic power of a test is related to the prevalence of the index disorder being tested (Baldessarini et al. 1983). Prevalence can also be regarded as the pretest probability of an individual's having the index disorder in a given population. We approach patients based on the population from which they come with a certain knowledge of the probability that the individual will have a personality disorder. Although the prevalence of personality disorders is relatively low in the general population, the prevalence increases in certain clinical populations and in certain clinical settings. For example, we would expect the lowest prevalence of personality disorders to be found in the community, slightly higher rates in outpatients, still higher rates in inpatient psychiatric settings, and the highest rates in prisons and mental institutions.

As we interview the patient, we gain further knowledge of the individual, which then raises the suspicion (and so the pretest probability) of the presence of a specific personality disorder. A test (our optimal criterion) is of greatest diagnostic value when the pretest likelihood is greater than 50/50 (greater than 50% probability) that the patient has the personality disorder (Sackett et al. 1991). This means that the clinician must have a high index of suspicion that the patient has a particular personality disorder before asking about the optimal criterion during the clinical interview. In this way, the clinician can maximize the power of the test.

It must also be borne in mind that all tests are vulnerable to false-positive results, and a positive result of any test only has the effect of increasing the posttest probability that the patient has a personality disorder. The prudent clinician would, therefore, use the optimal criterion test only as an aid to make a more accurate Axis II diagnosis.

Step 1: Be Aware of the Factors That Raise the Suspicion of the Presence of One Personality Disorder Over Another

To take the first step in determining which specific personality disorder to consider, the clinician should review the factors that affect the prevalence or pretest probability of one personality disorder over another. The following factors should be remembered:

- The prevalence of the personality disorder in the general population should be considered. For example, dependent personality disorder is fairly prevalent in community samples (7%), whereas narcissistic personality disorder is uncommonly diagnosed (< 0.5%).
- The setting in which the patient is seen is also important. The prevalence of personality disorders is higher in inpatient than in outpatient psychiatric settings and higher in outpatient settings than in a family practice setting.
- How the patient came to the clinician's attention may be of relevance. As stated in Chapter 1, patients with egodystonic disorders may bring themselves in for help, whereas patients with egosyntonic disorders more often present at the insistence of someone in their environment.
- The patient should be assessed for the presence of an Axis I disorder. The presence of certain Axis I disorders is associated with specific personality disorders.
- Evidence of a family history of psychiatric illness should be reviewed with the patient or family member. The clinician should ask about a history of psychiatric illness in the family and the occurrence of personality traits in family members. Personality disorders tend to run in families, and schizotypal and paranoid personality disorders are found with increased frequency in the family members of schizophrenic and paranoid psychotic patients (Siever and Davis 1991).
- Particular attention should be paid to the developmental history for certain risk factors that may be associated with specific personality disorders. For example, childhood shyness, fears of strangers, and novel situations may raise the clinician's suspicion that a person has avoidant personality disorder. Borderline personality disorder has been related to a history of childhood sexual abuse (Links and van Reekum 1993).
- A recurrent pattern of interpersonal interactions should be sought when the patient's social history is reviewed.
- Consider how severely and pervasively the patient's functioning is affected by the personality disorder. The personality disorders may be ordered in a hierarchical manner based on their

severity. Gunderson et al. (1991a) used an analogy to geology to explain the different levels of severity of personality disorders. A rock formation with structural faults will break apart in a predictable manner. If the faults are deep or more severe, or originate at the very base of the structure, the rock formation will break apart in a predictable but limited way. Personality disorders that are considered to be more severe have deeper "faults" originating from early developmental failure, have more profound neurophysiological changes, are more related to Axis I disorders, and show less variation from one situation to another.

Gunderson considered schizotypal, paranoid, narcissistic, antisocial, and borderline personality disorders to be the more severe disorders. If the faults are close to the surface, leaving the underlying structure intact, then the rock formation will break apart with much greater variation and less predictability. From this analogy, compulsive, histrionic, avoidant, and dependent personality disorders are considered to be less severe and more likely to extend into variations of normal personality. This hierarchy of personality disorders can be useful clinically. If more than one disorder is suspected, it is useful to focus on the disorder that may be considered more severe and more likely to lead to dysfunction.

Step 2: Use the Optimal Criterion During the Clinical Interview

After considering all these factors, the clinician will often find that one particular disorder is suspected (i.e., the pretest probability for this disorder is highest). The next step is to look for evidence to establish the optimal criterion during the clinical interview. We now review each of the personality disorders from DSM-IV, highlighting their prevalence in various settings, their associations with Axis I disorders, and their co-occurrence with other Axis II disorders. We also indicate the optimal criterion for each personality disorder diagnosis and our rationale for choosing the particular item. (Data on individual criteria were provided by

Dr. B. Pfohl, Co-occurrence and Diagnostic Efficiency Statistics; unpublished raw data, February 1993.)

Antisocial Personality Disorder

The rate of antisocial personality disorder in the general population is 1.9%–2.9% (Weissman 1993). In community samples, 3% of males and 1% of females receive this diagnosis (American Psychiatric Association 1994). Prevalence rates of antisocial personality disorder will be much higher in substance abuse treatment settings and forensic services. Axis I diagnoses that may occur with antisocial personality disorder include major depression, anxiety disorders, substance abuse/dependence, and somatization disorder (American Psychiatric Association 1994). The Axis I diagnosis that commonly blurs with the diagnosis of antisocial personality disorder is substance abuse/dependence. It is difficult, and often requires careful history taking from collateral sources, to distinguish substance abuse/dependence and secondary antisocial behaviors from antisocial personality disorder with secondary substance abuse/dependence.

To diagnose antisocial personality disorder, the interviewer needs to establish that the individual is age 18 years or older and has a history of conduct disorder traits before age 15. This history helps establish the behaviors as pervasive and maladaptive. Exploration of the early social and developmental history can also help the clinician differentiate between substance dependence with secondary antisocial behavior and substance dependence as a manifestation of antisocial personality disorder.

Antisocial personality disorder is an excellent example of the kind of personality disorder that is generally egosyntonic and might come to a clinician's attention because of others in the patient's environment or, if on the patient's own volition, for secondary gain. As stated, a collateral history is important in these patients to confirm the information obtained from them.

Most of the DSM-IV criteria describe criminal or delinquent behavior (Table 2–2). No single criterion is believed to be prototypical. Criterion 2, "deceitfulness," has the highest PPV. Irrespective of this, however, it is likely that the best way to establish a diagnosis of antisocial personality disorder in the clinical inter-

Table 2–2.   DSM-IV diagnostic criteria for 301.7 antisocial personality disorder

A. There is a pervasive pattern of disregard for and violation of the
    rights of others occurring since age 15 years, as indicated by three
    (or more) of the following:
    (1) failure to conform to social norms with respect to lawful be-
         haviors as indicated by repeatedly performing acts that are
         grounds for arrest
    (2) deceitfulness, as indicated by repeated lying, use of ali-
         ases, or conning others for personal profit or pleasure
    (3) impulsivity or failure to plan ahead
    (4) irritability and aggressiveness, as indicated by repeated
         physical fights or assaults
    (5) reckless disregard for safety of self or others
    (6) consistent irresponsibility, as indicated by repeated failure
         to sustain consistent work behavior or honor financial obli-
         gations
    (7) lack of remorse, as indicated by being indifferent to or ra-
         tionalizing having hurt, mistreated, or stolen from another

B. The individual is at least age 18 years.

C. There is evidence of conduct disorder with onset before age 15
    years.

D. The occurrence of antisocial behavior is not exclusively during the
    course of schizophrenia or a manic episode.

Source.   Reprinted from American Psychiatric Association: *Diagnostic and
Statistical Manual of Mental Disorders,* 4th Edition. Washington, DC, American
Psychiatric Association, 1994, pp. 649–650. Used with permission.

view is to explore the patient's social and personal history for
criminal, aggressive, impulsive, and irresponsible behaviors. An
attempt should be made to determine whether the antisocial behaviors preceded the onset of substance abuse and whether they
have been present since childhood. Other personality disorders
that may occur along with antisocial personality disorder include
narcissistic, histrionic, paranoid, and borderline personality disorders (American Psychiatric Association 1994).

Avoidant Personality Disorder

The prevalence of avoidant personality disorder in the general population ranges from 0.4% to 1.3% (Weissman 1993). Approximately 10% of outpatients seen in mental health clinics meet the criteria for avoidant personality disorder (American Psychiatric Association 1994). Avoidant personality disorder is diagnosed with similar frequency in men and women (American Psychiatric Association 1994). The Axis I diagnosis that most commonly occurs with or is confused with avoidant personality disorder is social phobia. In fact, some experts consider the disorders to be the same condition (American Psychiatric Association 1994). Other Axis I diagnoses that occur with avoidant personality disorder include major depression and posttraumatic stress disorder (American Psychiatric Association 1994).

The DSM-IV criterion with the highest PPV is criterion 1, "avoids occupational activities that involve significant interpersonal contact, because of fears of criticism, disapproval, or rejection" (Table 2–3). This trait is behaviorally based and can easily be examined in the social and personal history. As well as being behavioral, this trait is prototypical in that it encompasses a number of the other traits, such as those reflected in criteria 2 and 7, which also have high PPVs. Therefore, the optimal criterion to explore when avoidant personality disorder is suspected is criterion 1.

To distinguish avoidant personality disorder from schizoid personality disorder, the clinician must recall that individuals with avoidant personality disorder have an overt and objectively observable desire for a relationship and experience interpersonal anxiety when involved in a relationship. The patient with schizoid personality disorder has overt and objectively observed interpersonal indifference and exhibits little interest in being part of a relationship. Another personality disorder commonly misdiagnosed as avoidant is dependent personality disorder. Individuals with dependent personality disorder, in contrast to avoidant individuals, seek to be taken care of in relationships, whereas patients with avoidant personality disorder wish to avoid humiliation or rejection in relationships (American Psychiatric Association 1994). Other personality disorders that frequently coexist with avoidant personality disorder include borderline, paranoid,

Table 2–3. DSM-IV diagnostic criteria for 301.82 avoidant personality disorder

A pervasive pattern of social inhibition, feelings of inadequacy, and hypersensitivity to negative evaluation, beginning by early adulthood and present in a variety of contexts, as indicated by four (or more) of the following:

(1) avoids occupational activities that involve significant interpersonal contact, because of fears of criticism, disapproval, or rejection

(2) is unwilling to get involved with people unless certain of being liked

(3) shows restraint within intimate relationships because of the fear of being shamed or ridiculed

(4) is preoccupied with being criticized or rejected in social situations

(5) is inhibited in new interpersonal situations because of feelings of inadequacy

(6) views self as socially inept, personally unappealing, or inferior to others

(7) is unusually reluctant to take personal risks or to engage in any new activities because they may prove embarrassing

Source. Reprinted from American Psychiatric Association: *Diagnostic and Statistical Manual of Mental Disorders,* 4th Edition. Washington, DC, American Psychiatric Association, 1994, pp. 664–665. Used with permission.

and schizotypal personality disorders (American Psychiatric Association 1994).

Borderline Personality Disorder

The prevalence of borderline personality disorder in the general population is roughly 1%–2% (Swartz et al. 1990). Approximately 8%–10% of outpatients and 15% of inpatients meet criteria for borderline personality disorder (Links 1987). Borderline personality disorder is about three to four times more commonly diagnosed in women than in men (American Psychiatric Association 1994). The Axis I diagnoses that often occur with borderline personality disorder include major depression, substance abuse disorders, generalized anxiety disorder, posttraumatic stress disorder, phobias, cyclothymia, eating disorders, and attention-deficit hyperactivity disorder (American Psychiatric Association 1994; Gunderson et al. 1991c).

The criterion with the highest PPV is criterion 1, "frantic efforts to avoid real or imagined abandonment" (Table 2–4). The criterion with the second highest PPV is criterion 5, "recurrent suicidal behavior, gestures, or threats, or self-mutilating behavior." Individuals with borderline personality disorder often respond to abandonment with a variety of self-destructive acts (e.g., overdosing or wrist-slashing). However, their response may

Table 2–4.   DSM-IV diagnostic criteria for 301.83 borderline personality disorder

A pervasive pattern of instability of interpersonal relationships, self-image, and affects, and marked impulsivity beginning by early adulthood and present in a variety of contexts, as indicated by five (or more) of the following:

(1) frantic efforts to avoid real or imagined abandonment.
     Note: Do not include suicidal or self-mutilating behavior covered in Criterion 5.
(2) a pattern of unstable and intense interpersonal relationships characterized by alternating between extremes of idealization and devaluation
(3) identity disturbance: markedly and persistently unstable self-image or sense of self
(4) impulsivity in at least two areas that are potentially self-damaging (e.g., spending, sex, substance abuse, reckless driving, binge eating). **Note:** Do not include suicidal or self-mutilating behavior covered in Criterion 5.
(5) recurrent suicidal behavior, gestures, or threats, or self-mutilating behavior
(6) affective instability due to a marked reactivity of mood (e.g., intense episodic dysphoria, irritability, or anxiety usually lasting a few hours and only rarely more than a few days)
(7) chronic feelings of emptiness
(8) inappropriate, intense anger or difficulty controlling anger (e.g., frequent displays of temper, constant anger, recurrent physical fights)
(9) transient, stress-related paranoid ideation or severe dissociative symptoms

Source. Reprinted from American Psychiatric Association: *Diagnostic and Statistical Manual of Mental Disorders,* 4th Edition. Washington, DC, American Psychiatric Association, 1994, p. 654. Used with permission.

also include other impulsive and self-destructive behaviors, such as substance abuse, promiscuity, binge eating, overspending, and reckless driving. These impulsive behaviors are included in criterion 4. Fear of abandonment can also create ambivalent feelings about relationships and interfere with the ability to have stable, enduring relationships (as per criterion 2). Anger and angry outbursts may predominate and may be triggered by real or imagined abandonment. Therefore, criterion 1 is prototypical in that it explains the behaviors described in criteria 2, 4, 5, and 8 and has the highest PPV. Criterion 1 is the optimal criterion.

The area to explore in the clinical interview with the suspected borderline patient is behavior and emotional response to real or perceived abandonment in the context of his or her relationships. Dysphoria, anger, and impulsive and self-destructive behaviors should be elicited in questioning about the history of past and current relationships.

Ten percent of patients with a diagnosis of borderline personality disorder meet criteria for the borderline diagnosis alone. The clinician must bear in mind that up to 90% of patients with a diagnosis of borderline personality disorder meet criteria for other personality disorders, including histrionic personality disorder, schizotypal personality disorder, avoidant personality disorder, and antisocial personality disorder (Pfohl and Blum 1991).

Dependent Personality Disorder

The prevalence of dependent personality disorder has been reported to be 1.6%–6.7% in the general population (Weissman 1993). This diagnosis is one of the most frequently reported personality disorders in patients in mental health clinics (American Psychiatric Association 1994). Studies in which structured assessments were used have reported prevalence rates to be similar in men and women (American Psychiatric Association 1994). Axis I diagnoses that might occur with dependent personality disorder include agoraphobia, posttraumatic stress disorder, generalized anxiety disorder, social phobia, and major depression (Hirschfeld et al. 1991).

The relatively low PPVs for dependent personality disorder make it difficult to choose a criterion on which to focus. Two dimensions have been identified as prototypical for dependent personality disorder: 1) attachment with emotional reliance on another person and 2) dependency as a result of a lack of social self-confidence (Hirschfeld et al. 1991). These two dimensions imply a need for reassurance and support through proximity to others. Criteria 1 and 2 have the highest PPVs (Table 2–5). Criterion 2 is more easily established from history or collateral reports and is prototypical because it addresses the two dimensions of "reliance and self-confidence." Therefore, the optimal criterion is criterion 2, "needs others to assume responsibility for most major areas of his or her life." Using this criterion, the clinician can further explore the individual's lack of self-confidence and the extent of his or her reliance on others to alleviate anxiety around

Table 2–5.   DSM-IV diagnostic criteria for 301.6 dependent personality disorder

A pervasive and excessive need to be taken care of that leads to submissive and clinging behavior and fears of separation, beginning by early adulthood and present in a variety of contexts, as indicated by five (or more) of the following:

(1) has difficulty making everyday decisions without an excessive amount of advice and reassurance from others

(2) needs others to assume responsibility for most major areas of his or her life

(3) has difficulty expressing disagreement with others because of fear of loss of support or approval. **Note:**   Do not include realistic fears of retribution.

(4) has difficulty initiating projects or doing things on his or her own (because of a lack of self-confidence in judgment or abilities rather than a lack of motivation or energy)

(5) goes to excessive lengths to obtain nurturance and support from others, to the point of volunteering to do things that are unpleasant

(6) feels uncomfortable or helpless when alone because of exaggerated fears of being unable to care for himself or herself

(7) urgently seeks another relationship as a source of care and support when a close relationship ends

(8) is unrealistically preoccupied with fears of being left to take care of himself or herself

Source.   Reprinted from American Psychiatric Association: *Diagnostic and Statistical Manual of Mental Disorders,* 4th Edition. Washington, DC, American Psychiatric Association, 1994, pp. 668–669. Used with permission.

making decisions while maintaining a subservient position in the relationship. Other personality disorders that may overlap or co-exist with dependent personality disorder include borderline, avoidant, and histrionic personality disorders.

Histrionic Personality Disorder

The prevalence of histrionic personality disorder in the general population is 1.3%–3.0% (Weissman 1993). When structured assessments are used, several studies report equivalent prevalence rates among men and women (American Psychiatric Association 1994). Axis I diagnoses that can occur with histrionic personality disorder include major depression, conversion disorder, and somatization disorder (American Psychiatric Association 1994).

An examination of the DSM-IV criteria for histrionic personality disorder (Table 2–6) reveals that criterion 2, "interaction with others is often characterized by inappropriate sexually seductive

Table 2–6. DSM-IV diagnostic criteria for 301.50 histrionic personality disorder

A pervasive pattern of excessive emotionality and attention seeking, beginning by early adulthood and present in a variety of contexts, as indicated by five (or more) of the following:

(1) is uncomfortable in situations in which he or she is not the center of attention
(2) interaction with others is often characterized by inappropriate sexually seductive or provocative behavior
(3) displays rapidly shifting and shallow expression of emotions
(4) consistently uses physical appearance to draw attention to self
(5) has a style of speech that is excessively impressionistic and lacking in detail
(6) shows self-dramatization, theatricality, and exaggerated expression of emotion
(7) is suggestible, i.e., easily influenced by others or circumstances
(8) considers relationships to be more intimate than they actually are

Source. Reprinted from American Psychiatric Association: *Diagnostic and Statistical Manual of Mental Disorders,* 4th Edition. Washington, DC, American Psychiatric Association, 1994, pp. 657–658. Used with permission.

or provocative behavior," and criterion 1, "is uncomfortable in situations in which he or she is not the center of attention," have the highest PPVs. Criterion 1 can be seen as prototypical because the discomfort that these individuals feel when they are not the center of attention may result in various attention-seeking behaviors. To remain the center of attention, the individual might engage in the behaviors reflected in criteria 4, 5, and 6, which include theatrical verbal and emotional expression. Thus, criterion 1 is considered the optimal criterion. This criterion, although not having the highest PPV, is prototypical and is related to most of the behaviors characteristic of histrionic personality disorder.

In the interview, the clinician should explore the individual's emotional and behavioral response to the loss of feeling the center of attention, focusing on sexually seductiveness, dramatic exaggerated emotional expression, and the use of physical appearance to draw attention to oneself.

As mentioned, there is a high co-occurrence of borderline personality disorder in patients with histrionic personality disorder. Other personality disorders that coexist with histrionic personality disorder are narcissistic, antisocial, and dependent personality disorders (American Psychiatric Association 1994; Pfohl 1991).

Narcissistic Personality Disorder

The prevalence of narcissistic personality disorder is relatively low in the general population, 0.4% (Weissman 1993). The prevalence in clinical populations may range from 2% to 16%, and more than half of diagnosed patients are male (American Psychiatric Association 1994). Axis I disorders that may occur with narcissistic personality disorder include major depression, bipolar affective disorder, anorexia nervosa, substance abuse/dependence, and dysthymia (American Psychiatric Association 1994).

The diagnostic category of narcissistic personality disorder is of interest to many from a psychodynamic perspective. The central descriptors of this personality disorder are derived from psychoanalytic theory, and as a result the criteria tend to be more subjective than for other personality disorders. The clinician must rely on the individual's reporting of his or her subjective experiences.

The essential feature of narcissistic personality disorder appears to be "grandiosity" (Gunderson et al. 1991b). Many of the other features are conceptually related to the patient's sense of self-importance (Table 2–7). Criterion 1, "has a grandiose sense of self-importance," has the second highest PPV after criterion 6, "is interpersonally exploitative." With this grandiose view, the individual may have expectations of his or her environment and future that relate to other criteria, such as 2, 3, 4, and 5. Therefore, we may consider criterion 1 as prototypical and as the optimal criterion for narcissistic personality disorder. The clinician should ask the patient to describe himself or herself and characterize his or her own strengths and weaknesses.

Individuals with narcissistic personality disorder will also

Table 2–7. DSM-IV diagnostic criteria for 301.81 narcissistic personality disorder

A pervasive pattern of grandiosity (in fantasy or behavior), need for admiration, and lack of empathy, beginning by early adulthood and present in a variety of contexts, as indicated by five (or more) of the following:

(1) has a grandiose sense of self-importance (e.g., exaggerates achievements and talents, expects to be recognized as superior without commensurate achievements)

(2) is preoccupied with fantasies of unlimited success, power, brilliance, beauty, or ideal love

(3) believes that he or she is "special" and unique and can only be understood by, or should associate with, other special or high-status people (or institutions)

(4) requires excessive admiration

(5) has a sense of entitlement, i.e., unreasonable expectations of especially favorable treatment or automatic compliance with his or her expectations

(6) is interpersonally exploitative, i.e., takes advantage of others to achieve his or her own ends

(7) lacks empathy: is unwilling to recognize or identify with the feelings and needs of others

(8) is often envious of others or believes that others are envious of him or her

(9) shows arrogant, haughty behaviors or attitudes

Source. Reprinted from American Psychiatric Association: *Diagnostic and Statistical Manual of Mental Disorders,* 4th Edition. Washington, DC, American Psychiatric Association, 1994, p. 661. Used with permission.

often meet criteria for antisocial, borderline, paranoid, and histrionic personality disorders (American Psychiatric Association 1994).

Obsessive-Compulsive Personality Disorder

The prevalence of obsessive-compulsive personality disorder is 1.7%–6.4% in the general population (Weissman 1993). Up to 10% of patients in mental health clinics meet the criteria for this disorder, and twice as many males as females receive a diagnosis of obsessive-compulsive personality disorder (American Psychiatric Association 1994).

There is no etiological relation between obsessive-compulsive personality disorder and obsessive-compulsive disorder, and the co-occurrence of these disorders has not been demonstrated consistently (American Psychiatric Association 1994). Other Axis I disorders that might occur with obsessive-compulsive personality disorder are major depression and anxiety disorders (American Psychiatric Association 1994).

The Lazare-Klerman Trait Scale (LKTS), in which psychoanalytically derived traits are used, lists the following as most characteristic of obsessive-compulsive personality disorder (Pfohl and Blum 1991):

- Orderliness
- Strong superego
- Perseverance
- Obstinacy
- Rigidity
- Rejection of others
- Parsimony
- Emotional constriction

The DSM criteria for obsessive-compulsive personality disorder that have the highest PPVs are criterion 2, "shows perfectionism that interferes with task completion," and criterion 4, "overconscientious, scrupulous, and inflexible about matters of morality, ethics, and values." These criteria appear to be prototypical in that they capture the LKTS characteristic traits. The criterion to explore and to use as the optimal criterion when ob-

Table 2–8. DSM-IV diagnostic criteria for 301.4 obsessive-compulsive personality disorder

A pervasive pattern of preoccupation with orderliness, perfectionism, and mental and interpersonal control, at the expense of flexibility, openness, and efficiency, beginning by early adulthood and present in a variety of contexts, as indicated by four (or more) of the following:
   (1) is preoccupied with details, rules, lists, order, organization, or schedules to the extent that the major point of the activity is lost
   (2) shows perfectionism that interferes with task completion (e.g., is unable to complete a project because his or her own overly strict standards are not met)
   (3) is excessively devoted to work and productivity to the exclusion of leisure activities and friendships (not accounted for by obvious economic necessity)
   (4) is overconscientious, scrupulous, and inflexible about matters of morality, ethics, or values (not accounted for by cultural or religious identification)
   (5) is unable to discard worn-out or worthless objects even when they have no sentimental value
   (6) is reluctant to delegate tasks or to work with others unless they submit to exactly his or her way of doing things
   (7) adopts a miserly spending style toward both self and others; money is viewed as something to be hoarded for future catastrophes
   (8) shows rigidity and stubbornness

Source. Reprinted from American Psychiatric Association: *Diagnostic and Statistical Manual of Mental Disorders,* 4th Edition. Washington, DC, American Psychiatric Association, 1994, pp. 672–673. Used with permission.

sessive-compulsive personality disorder is suspected is criterion 2, "shows perfectionism that interferes with task completion, e.g., is unable to complete a project because his or her own overly strict standards are not met" (Table 2–8). Overlap with other personality disorders requires more study.

Paranoid Personality Disorder

The prevalence of paranoid personality disorder in the general population is 0.4%–1.8% (Weissman 1993). DSM-IV indicates that the disorder may be diagnosed in 10%–30% of inpatients and up to 10% of outpatients from mental health clinics. The Axis I disorders associated with paranoid personality disorder are delusional disorder, schizophrenia, major depression, obsessive-compulsive disorder, and agoraphobia without panic attacks (American Psychiatric Association 1994).

The criterion with the highest PPV is criterion 1 (Table 2–9). Although not behavioral, this criterion is prototypical in that it

Table 2–9.   DSM-IV diagnostic criteria for 301.0 paranoid personality disorder

A. A pervasive distrust and suspiciousness of others such that their motives are interpreted as malevolent, beginning by early adulthood and present in a variety of contexts, as indicated by four (or more) of the following:
    (1) suspects, without sufficient basis, that others are exploiting, harming, or deceiving him or her
    (2) is preoccupied with unjustified doubts about the loyalty or trustworthiness of friends or associates
    (3) is reluctant to confide in others because of unwarranted fear that the information will be used maliciously against him or her
    (4) reads hidden demeaning or threatening meanings into benign remarks or events
    (5) persistently bears grudges, i.e., is unforgiving of insults, injuries, or slights
    (6) perceives attacks on his or her character or reputation that are not apparent to others and is quick to react angrily or to counterattack
    (7) has recurrent suspicions, without justification, regarding fidelity of spouse or sexual partner

B. Does not occur exclusively during the course of schizophrenia, a mood disorder with psychotic features, or another psychotic disorder and is not due to the direct physiological effects of a general medical condition.
    Note: If criteria are met prior to the onset of schizophrenia, add "premorbid," e.g., "paranoid personality disorder (premorbid)."

Source.   Reprinted from American Psychiatric Association: *Diagnostic and Statistical Manual of Mental Disorders,* 4th Edition. Washington, DC, American Psychiatric Association, 1994, pp. 637–638. Used with permission.

relates to the behaviors and attitudes described by criteria 3, 4, and 7 that may be elicited in taking a full history of the patient's relationships. Therefore, criterion 1, "suspects, without sufficient basis, that others are exploiting, harming, or deceiving him or her," and its behavioral manifestations of suspiciousness should increase the probability of making a correct diagnosis of paranoid personality disorder and can be considered the optimal criterion. Narcissistic, borderline, avoidant, schizotypal, and schizoid personality disorders can co-occur with paranoid personality disorder.

Schizoid Personality Disorder

The prevalence of schizoid personality disorder in the general population is 0.4%–0.9% (Weissman 1993). The disorder is believed to be uncommon in clinical settings and is diagnosed more often in men than in women (American Psychiatric Association 1994). The term *schizoid* describes a tendency for these individuals to withdraw from the external world with emotional bluntness resembling the negative symptoms of schizophrenia. The negative symptoms of schizophrenia are associated with increased heritability of schizophrenia and suggest a genetic link between schizophrenia and schizoid personality disorder, although the nature of this association is not clear (Kalus et al. 1991). When schizoid personality disorder is being diagnosed, schizophrenia and delusional disorder should always be considered either as possibly coexistent or in the differential diagnosis (American Psychiatric Association 1994).

The criterion with the highest PPV is criterion 1, "neither desires nor enjoys close relationships, including being part of a family" (Table 2–10). By exploring for this criterion, the clinician will elicit information about other aspects of the diagnosis, such as choosing solitary activities, having no close friends, and showing little interest in having sexual experiences with another person. Therefore, criterion 1 is considered prototypical and should be considered as the optimal criterion.

Other personality disorders that coexist with schizoid personality disorder are schizotypal, paranoid, and avoidant personality disorders.

Table 2–10.   DSM-IV diagnostic criteria for 301.20 schizoid personality disorder

A. A pervasive pattern of detachment from social relationships and a restricted range of expression of emotions in interpersonal settings, beginning by early adulthood and present in a variety of contexts, as indicated by four (or more) of the following:

    (1) neither desires nor enjoys close relationships, including being part of a family

    (2) almost always chooses solitary activities

    (3) has little, if any, interest in having sexual experiences with another person

    (4) takes pleasure in few, if any, activities

    (5) lacks close friends or confidants other than first-degree relatives

    (6) appears indifferent to the praise or criticism of others

    (7) shows emotional coldness, detachment, or flattened affectivity

B. Does not occur exclusively during the course of schizophrenia, a mood disorder with psychotic features, another psychotic disorder, or a pervasive developmental disorder and is not due to the direct physiological effects of a general medical condition.

    Note: If criteria are met prior to the onset of schizophrenia, add "premorbid," e.g., "schizoid personality disorder (premorbid)."

Source.   Reprinted from American Psychiatric Association: *Diagnostic and Statistical Manual of Mental Disorders,* 4th Edition. Washington, DC, American Psychiatric Association, 1994, p. 641. Used with permission.

Schizotypal Personality Disorder

The prevalence of schizotypal personality disorder in the general population is 3%–5.6% (Weissman 1993). Schizotypal personality disorder was added to DSM-III in an attempt to describe individuals that presented with mild psychotic-like features, social isolation, and poor rapport. Family members with relatives diagnosed with schizophrenia were found to have biological, interpersonal, and cognitive vulnerabilities that were similar to but milder than those found in individuals with schizophrenia (Siever et al. 1991). As a result, the diagnosis is considered by some as part of the spectrum of schizophrenic disorders and has been considered as an Axis I rather than an Axis II diagnosis. Nevertheless, it is currently regarded as "the only personality disorder to be defined empirically on the basis of a genetic relationship to an Axis I disorder" (Siever et al. 1991, p. 180). Axis I disorders that can occur with schizotypal personality disorder include brief psychotic disorder, schizophreniform disorder, delusional disorder, schizophrenia, or, most commonly, major depression (American Psychiatric Association 1994).

Table 2–11. DSM-IV diagnostic criteria for 301.22 schizotypal personality disorder

A. A pervasive pattern of social and interpersonal deficits marked by acute discomfort with, and reduced capacity for, close relationships as well as by cognitive or perceptual distortions and eccentricities of behavior, beginning by early adulthood and present in a variety of contexts, as indicated by five (or more) of the following:
    (1) ideas of reference (excluding delusions of reference)
    (2) odd beliefs or magical thinking that influences behavior and is inconsistent with subcultural norms (e.g., superstitiousness, belief in clairvoyance, telepathy, or "sixth sense"; in children and adolescents, bizarre fantasies or preoccupations)
    (3) unusual perceptual experiences, including bodily illusions
    (4) odd thinking and speech (e.g., vague, circumstantial, metaphorical, overelaborate, or stereotyped)
    (5) suspiciousness or paranoid ideation
    (6) inappropriate or constricted affect
    (7) behavior or appearance that is odd, eccentric, or peculiar
    (8) lack of close friends or confidants other than first-degree relatives
    (9) excessive social anxiety that does not diminish with familiarity and tends to be associated with paranoid fears rather than negative judgments about self

B. Does not occur exclusively during the course of schizophrenia, a mood disorder with psychotic features, another psychotic disorder, or a pervasive developmental disorder.
    Note: If criteria are met prior to the onset of schizophrenia, add "premorbid," e.g., "schizotypal personality disorder (premorbid)."

Source. Reprinted from American Psychiatric Association: *Diagnostic and Statistical Manual of Mental Disorders,* 4th Edition. Washington, DC, American Psychiatric Association, 1994, p. 645. Used with permission.

Many researchers agree that the central disturbances in patients with schizotypal personality disorder are social withdrawal, odd or eccentric speech and behavior, and paranoid ideation (Siever et al. 1991). In regard to DSM-IV criteria for schizotypal personality disorder (Table 2–11), these central disturbances are addressed by criteria 4, 5, 7, and 9, which also have the highest PPVs. In addition, these criteria relate to components assessed from the mental status examination. Thus, criterion 4, "odd thinking and speech," and criterion 7, "behavior or appearance that is odd, eccentric, or peculiar," can be regarded together as the optimal criteria. The clinician confronted with a patient with persistent odd, inappropriate behavior, appearance, and speech or thoughts and in whom schizophrenia has been ruled out may suspect schizotypal personality disorder.

Schizotypal personality disorder has psychotic-like features that can be confused with those found in borderline personality disorder. The features of social inappropriateness and withdrawal are similar to the features of schizoid personality disorder. Therefore, the other personality disorders that overlap with schizotypal personality disorder are borderline, schizoid, paranoid, and avoidant personality disorders (American Psychiatric Association 1994).

Step 3: Apply Full DSM-IV Criteria to Confirm the Diagnosis

After the clinical interview has been completed, the clinician should attempt to confirm the personality disorder diagnosis by reviewing the full criteria from DSM-IV for the specific diagnosis. If the diagnosis from the clinical interview is confirmed, the clinician should make a mental note of those features that first raised suspicions about the diagnosis. Experienced clinicians characteristically can rapidly develop diagnostic hypotheses based on previous encounters with similar patients, which then can be tested during the clinical interview using the optimal criterion.

If the clinician is unable to confirm the personality disorder diagnosis after reviewing the full criteria set, then several steps should be considered. A patient with an acute symptom disorder will be difficult to assess for personality disorder diagnoses. The

Axis II diagnosis may appropriately be deferred until the symptoms of the acute disorder are diminished. During the acute state, most clinicians are likely to overdiagnose personality disorders, and patients will overendorse personality pathology (Zimmerman 1994). The clinician may seek collateral information from family or friends about the patient's personality features. However, research findings indicate that agreement between the patient's report and the informant are often poor (Zimmerman 1994), and it can be difficult to reconcile the different reports. Zimmerman (1994) suggested that the patient's report may be utilized for information about affective or cognitive aspects of personality, whereas the informant may be more reliable in characterizing the patient's interpersonal and behavioral functioning.

The clinician may attempt to confirm the diagnosis with psychological tests. (This approach to diagnosis is discussed in detail in Chapter 3.) Structured diagnostic interviews are available for making Axis II diagnoses. These interviews generally are much more reliable in that two clinicians are more likely to agree with each other about the diagnosis when structured rather than clinical interviews are used. However, these interviews are time-consuming to administer, require some training and practice with the particular procedure, and necessitate an experienced clinician to carry out the interview (Zimmerman 1994). The four major interviews currently available are all based on DSM-III-R criteria:

1. International Personality Disorder Examination (Loranger et al. 1994)
2. Structured Interview for DSM-III-R Personality Disorders (Stangl et al. 1985)
3. The Diagnostic Interview for Personality Disorders (Zanarini et al. 1987)
4. Structured Clinical Interview for DSM-III-R (SCID) (Spitzer et al. 1990; Williams et al. 1992)

If the clinician is still uncertain about making a specific personality disorder diagnosis, then he or she should be patient and await future opportunities to observe the patient. Observing the patient over time and in different contexts can assist in making specific personality disorder diagnoses.

Conclusion

This chapter identifies three steps for the clinician to follow when assessing a patient for a specific personality disorder diagnosis. Although these steps provide for a more systematic assessment of patients on the basis of the clinical interview, the diagnosis of personality disorders remains more an art than a science. Like other aspects of clinical practice, the diagnosis of personality disorders requires a sound knowledge of the disorders, a systematic method of evaluation, and extensive experience with patients with personality disorders to develop an expertise in this area of clinical assessment.

References

American Psychiatric Association: Diagnostic and Statistical Manual of Mental Disorders, 3rd Edition. Washington, DC, American Psychiatric Association, 1980

American Psychiatric Association: Diagnostic and Statistical Manual of Mental Disorders, 3rd Edition, Revised. Washington, DC, American Psychiatric Association, 1987

American Psychiatric Association: Diagnostic Statistical Manual of Mental Disorders, 4th Edition. Washington, DC, American Psychiatric Association, 1994

Baldessarini R, Finkelstein S, Arana G: The predictive power of diagnostic tests and the effect of prevalence on illness. Arch Gen Psychiatry 40:569–573, 1983

Gunderson JG, Links PS, Reich JH: Competing models of personality disorders. Journal of Personality Disorders 5:60–68, 1991a

Gunderson J, Rossingstam E, Smith E: Narcissistic personality disorder: a review of the data of DSM-III-R descriptions. Journal of Personality Disorders 5:167–172, 1991b

Gunderson J, Zanarini M, Cassandra L: Borderline personality disorder: a review of the data on DSM-III-R descriptions. Journal of Personality Disorders 5:340–352, 1991c

Hirschfeld R, Shea M, Weise R: Dependent personality disorder: perspectives for DSM-IV. Journal of Personality Disorders 5:135–149, 1991

Kalus O, Bernstein P, Siever L: Schizoid personality disorder: a review of current status for DSM-IV. Journal of Personality Disorders 7:43–52, 1991

Links PS: Borderline personality disorder: validity revisited. Psychiatric Medicine 4:25–37, 1987

Links PS, van Reekum R: Childhood sexual abuse, parental impairment and the development of borderline personality disorder. Can J Psychiatry 38:472–474, 1993

Loranger AW, Sartorius N, Andreoli A, et al: The International Personality Disorder Examination: The World Health Organization/Alcohol, Drug Abuse, and Mental Health Administration International Pilot Study of Personality Disorders. Arch Gen Psychiatry 51:215–224, 1994

Perry JC: Challenges in validating personality disorders: beyond description. Journal of Personality Disorders 4:273–289, 1990

Pfohl B: Histrionic personality disorder: a review of available data and recommendations for DSM-IV. Journal of Personality Disorders 5:150–166, 1991

Pfohl B, Blum N: Obsessive compulsive personality disorder: a review for DSM-IV. Journal of Personality Disorders 5:363–375, 1991

Sackett DL, Haynes B, Tugwell D: Clinical Epidemiology: A Basic Science for Clinical Medicine, 2nd Edition. Boston, MA, Little, Brown, 1991

Siever LJ, Davis KL: A psychobiological perspective on the personality disorders. Am J Psychiatry 148:1647–1658, 1991

Siever L, Bernstein D, Silverman J: Schizotypal personality disorder: a review of its current status. Journal of Personality Disorders 5:178–193, 1991

Spitzer RL, Williams JBW, Gibbon M: User's Guide for the Structured Clinical Interview for DSM-III-R (SCID). Washington, DC, American Psychiatric Press, 1990

Stangl D, Pfohl B, Zimmerman M, et al: A structured interview for DSM-III personality disorders: a preliminary report. Arch Gen Psychiatry 42:591–596, 1985

Swartz M, Blazer D, George L, et al: Estimating the prevalence of borderline personality disorder in the community. Journal of Personality Disorders 4:257–272, 1990

Weissman M: The epidemiology of personality disorders: a 1990 update. Journal of Personality Disorders 7 (suppl):44–62, 1993

Widiger T, Frances A: The DSM-III personality disorders: perspectives from psychology. Arch Gen Psychiatry 42:615–623, 1985

Williams JBW, Gibbon M, First MB, et al: The Structured Clinical Interview for DSM-III-R (SCID), II: multisite test-retest reliability. Arch Gen Psychiatry 49:630–636, 1992

Zanarini M, Frankenburg FR, Chauncey DL, et al: The Diagnostic Interview for Personality Disorders: interrater and test-retest reliability. Compr Psychiatry 28:467–480, 1987

Zimmerman M: Diagnosing personality disorders: a review of issues and research methods. Arch Gen Psychiatry 51:225–245, 1994

CHAPTER 3

Use of Psychological Tests in the Diagnosis and Treatment of Personality Disorders

Jayne Patrick, Ph.D.

*P*sychological testing has been used as an adjunct to psychiatric diagnosis since the nineteenth century (Anastasi 1988). Psychological assessment of personality functioning dates back more than 70 years; the need for classification of military personnel during World War II constituted a major impetus for its development. Psychological assessment of personality functioning rests on the assumption that the thoughts, feelings, and behaviors expressed by each individual are indicative of characteristics that have developed over the span of his or her lifetime. Psychological testing thus addresses a broad range of interrelated personality features, including perceptions, emotions, cognitive processes, and interpersonal behaviors. In order to understand the development and use of psychological tests in the assessment of personality dysfunction, the concept of personality per se must first be briefly examined.

Personality develops from birth onward as an accumulation and consolidation of responses by the developing infant to the external environment and internal need states. A diagnosis of personality disorder tends to be made when a patient exhibits chronic, long-standing problems in interpersonal functioning that are relatively severe and resistant to change. Additional criteria for the diagnosis of personality disorder include early onset (adolescence or young adulthood), stability or persistence over time, pervasiveness (behavior affected in various contexts, such as family, work, and social situations), and disturbances in intrapsychic and interpersonal functioning (Hirschfeld 1993). Psychodynamic theories of personality dysfunction in particular emphasize the role of early childhood experiences in the development of adult character and psychopathology. Given the fact that personality pathology arises out of the interplay of environmental and constitutional factors from birth through adulthood, the understanding of the nature and degree of psychopathology in a given patient can be greatly enhanced by an awareness of the salient aspects of his or her developmental history.

Although infants basically share the same need states, there is considerable variability in the intensity and duration of these states and in each infant's capacity to seek out and respond to opportunities for the gratification of needs in his or her particular environment. This variability has its origins in constitutional (genetic) factors. Over time, the infant acquires a particular repertoire of internal and external responses to the environment. Gradually, a process of integration and consolidation takes place whereby this repertoire is transformed into what is regarded as personality structure.

Personality structure thus consists of a pattern of enduring traits or characteristic patterns of responding. Because personality structure is reflected in behavior, an individual's personality can be described and categorized by identifying typical behavior patterns. Personality traits thus represent the typical ways of thinking, feeling, and behaving that each individual has developed to meet both internal and external demands. Because these demands are often conflictual and contradictory, personality traits of necessity constitute compromise solutions.

Personality traits that serve the function of compromise solutions can be viewed simply as forms of learned behavior or, alternatively, as arising from internal mental processes. In the latter case, personality traits are a manifestation of an individual's wishes, prohibitions, and fears. For example, a common trait found in individuals with passive-aggressive personality disorders is a tendency to delay responding to requests from others.

Delayed compliance, as opposed to outright refusal, can serve simultaneously to express a number of contradictory internal responses, such as the following:

- Rebellion against perceived control or exploitation by others
- Denial of the desire to refuse a request or demand
- Hostility toward the individual making the request or demand
- Fear of punishment for hostile feelings and impulses
- Desire to be thought of as a cooperative (and thus worthwhile) person

When a compromise solution is sufficiently maladaptive and persists over time and across circumstances, it is said to constitute a personality disorder.

Role of Psychological Assessment

Psychological assessment serves both labor- and time-saving functions in the diagnosis and treatment of personality disorders. It also gives the practitioner access to sources of information that may lie outside of his or her particular area of expertise.

Personality assessment constitutes a tool that can assist in the evaluation and treatment process in various health care contexts. In both general and specialized medical practice, a referral for psychological testing is most often made when it is not possible to identify an organic basis for a patient's presenting problems or symptoms, when the symptom or complaint appears to be stress-related, or when the symptoms appear to have a psychosomatic component (e.g., migraine headaches, duodenal ulcer, chronic low back pain).

In psychiatric practice, referrals for psychological testing are typically made for both brief and in-depth assessments. In addition to a general clinical interview, patients referred for brief assessment complete one or more paper-and-pencil personality questionnaires. Test findings and interview data are then combined to address either a specific or a general referral question. For example, a brief psychometric assessment of personality functioning can serve the purpose of introducing a new patient to the treating psychiatrist, general practitioner, or mental health care worker. Used for this purpose, the assessment typically addresses the following issues:

- Differential diagnosis
- Current symptoms
- Coping resources
- Social functioning

A variety of specific problems or questions may give rise to an assessment referral. For example, psychological testing may be requested to assist in determining whether personality factors can account for a patient's lack of response to adequate trials of psychotropic medications, to determine whether a particular patient may be able to benefit from psychotherapy, or to select the most appropriate form of psychotherapy for a given patient.

The following case example illustrates the role of psychological testing in the diagnosis and treatment of personality disorders.

Case 1

Mr. A, a young businessman and recent university graduate, was referred by his family physician for a psychiatric consultation after he complained of panic attacks. Mr. A's first attack occurred en route to his graduation ceremonies and continued at a frequency of one to three times per week thereafter, accompanied by a significant increase in his general tension level. Mr. A's family physician tried treating him with a variety of anxiolytics. After 6 months had passed with only moderate success in reducing his tension and the frequency and intensity of his panic attacks, Mr. A was referred for a psychiatric consultation.

In his initial interviews with his psychiatrist, Mr. A appeared confident, intelligent, articulate, and cheerful. He disclosed the fact that he had just launched his own company, having had a phenomenally successful rise through the ranks of the firm he had joined after graduation. His tension was evident primarily in his constant shifting of his position in his seat and toying with his glasses and key chain. Mr. A acknowledged that his drive to succeed in his own business made for a stressful existence, but he denied feeling worried or depressed. He also stated that no area of his life constituted a source of dissatisfaction or concern for him. Exploration over a period of several sessions of the details of his family and social relationships and the state of his business affairs failed to suggest otherwise. When it was recommended that Mr. A attend a stress management course, he agreed without hesitation. Although he found the stress management techniques quite useful, he also continued to require a moderate dose of anxiolytic medication to keep his anxiety symptoms at a tolerable level. Throughout this period, Mr. A also continued to deny that he had experienced any significant disappointments in either his personal or professional life.

Approximately 6 months after his referral for psychiatric consultation, Mr. A began to complain of dysphoria secondary to his persistent feelings of nonspecific anxiety. Although he denied concerns about his job performance, concerns about the future success of his business ventures, or feelings of inadequacy or low self-esteem, he stated that his feelings of anxiety were beginning to exert an increasingly negative impact on all aspects of his life. His complaints centered on the fact that his levels of energy and drive were reduced and his capacity to experience pleasure had markedly diminished.

Mr. A was referred for psychological testing at this point to obtain further information on his personality structure and functioning. Testing was also done to determine whether he could benefit from psychotherapy that focused on understanding the deeper meanings of his symptoms or from a symptom relief approach focused on his anxiety.

Results of Mr. A's assessment proved to be quite revealing. (Test findings are described in more detail later in this chapter within the context of the specific tests employed.) Despite appearances to the contrary, Mr. A's assessment results indicated that he was emotionally very fragile. In addition to a generalized anxiety disorder, he exhibited marked paranoid and obsessive features within the context of severe personality pathology. Mr. A's test results also showed that he needed to perceive himself as being in control of most aspects of his life in order to maintain his contact with reality. Mr. A's own fear of decompensating into a psychotic state emerged as the root cause of his anxiety disorder.

A number of significant treatment implications evolved from these findings. Chief among these was the realization that any form of therapy that focused on removing the defenses that protected this patient from awareness of his emotional fragility would be contraindicated. In addition, the minor tranquilizers he had been prescribed could potentially precipitate a psychotic break by further undermining his defensive functioning.

Gaining an understanding of how personality factors may contribute to physical or emotional dysfunction is an important step in the evaluation and treatment process. Personality factors often contribute significantly to a lack of progress in treatment. As in the case example, psychological testing can help the practitioner understand the interrelationships between personality factors and the patient's presenting problems. Thus, the primary function of personality assessment is to use the information obtained from psychometric data to lay the foundation for further therapeutic intervention.

Psychometric approaches to the assessment of personality functioning include projective tests as well as empirically derived and objective personality assessment measures. All of these approaches entail the use of standardized procedures in which patients' responses can be compared with those of a normative group. Structured interview schedules are also standardized, but they differ from empirically derived and objective measures in that the latter are usually self-administered, with patients completing paper-and-pencil questionnaires (many of which can now be computer scored).

Like projective tests, structured interview schedules must be individually administered and generally require about 2 hours to complete and score. Extensive training and practice by those administering the test are necessary to ensure valid results. Structured interviews developed for the assessment of personality disorders offer greater diagnostic accuracy than do nonstandardized, less-structured interview procedures but are clearly quite labor intensive. However, they do not yield the in-depth information about personality dynamics that can be obtained from projective measures, which are also labor intensive. The convergent validity of categorically oriented structured interview measures has been demonstrated for specific instruments, but further research is needed to confirm the validity of dimensionally oriented structured interview measures. To date, structured interviews have been used primarily as research tools.

Categories of Personality Assessment Measures

Two major categories of psychometric tests are used to assess personality functioning and to diagnose personality disorders: projective and empirically derived measures. These categories reflect differences in both the test structure and the type of information provided by each kind of test.

Projective Tests

Projective testing evolved out of the observation that individuals tend to transpose salient aspects of their inner world onto external stimuli. Unlike objective tests, these measures are designed to elicit information that lies outside of a patient's conscious awareness and thus can bypass his or her denial of symptoms and behaviors. The use of projective measures also allows access to the individual's inner experience. Personality dysfunction (disorder) is expressed in symptoms and behaviors, and it is only through an awareness of an individual's inner experience that their meanings can be understood. If the meaning of a particular symptom or behavior lies outside of the individual's own awareness, knowledge of what it represents can assist the patient to bring it under conscious control. Likewise, knowledge of the underlying needs, wishes, and fears expressed through a particular symptom or behavior can lead to the development of alternative, less dysfunctional means of addressing these motivational states. It is in uncovering information of this nature, which lies at the root of personality dysfunction, that the primary value of projective testing resides.

The Rorschach test is the best known projective test (Aronow and Reznikoff 1976; Rabin 1968; Rapaport et al. 1945; Schafer 1954). It consists of a set of 10 ink blots printed on heavy cardboard squares. The ink blots only vaguely resemble aspects of physical reality (e.g., animals, faces, geographical features). As a result, the individual taking the test must call on internal resources (associations and imagination) to identify what each blot could represent. Of all psychological tests, therefore, the Rorschach is the least susceptible to conscious censoring processes. Rorschach responses are interpreted by taking into consideration data such as the images' content, sequence, and perceptual plausibility.

The Rorschach test has been used extensively in the diagnosis of personality dysfunction. The use of the Rorschach test in the assessment of patients who would now be diagnosed as having borderline personality disorders, for example, dates back almost 50 years. At that time, it was observed that patients with a diagnosis of latent schizophrenia, borderline psychosis, and schizophrenic character disorders had a unique Rorschach presentation, characterized by mild to moderate perceptual inaccuracy and blatantly "abnormal" content. Responses characteristic of these patients suggested that their normal repressive defenses were defective and readily breached when structure or familiarity was absent.

During the past 20 years, Rorschach research has focused more on the test presentation of borderline personality disorder than on any of the other personality disorders. In a review of Rorschach research on patients with borderline disorders, Singer (1977) reported that these patients produced bizarre, elaborated, idiosyncratic content on the Rorschach test but showed little evidence of thought disorder on more structured tests.

Rorschach protocols of borderline patients are often readily distinguishable from those of various other diagnostic groups (e.g., neurotic, "normal," and schizophrenic subjects, as well as those with other personality disorders) by the much higher frequency of 1) dramatic, negative, affective elaboration of precepts and 2) aggressive content. Examples include "two little girls with pony tails giving each other hateful looks"; "two ugly monsters tearing apart this poor creature in the middle"; and "an alien, with his mouth on top of his head, riding on a motorcycle." Such specific pathognomonic content, its pervasiveness, and the degree to which it deviates from normal percepts all assist the clinician to predict the suitability and outcome of psychotherapy and to make recommendations with respect to hospital treatment (Kwawer et al. 1980).

Various qualitative and quantitative features of the Rorschach test have also been shown to characterize other personality disorders. For example, test records of patients with histrionic and narcissistic personality disorders are similar to those of borderline patients in their predominance of emotionally charged imagery combined with evidence of poor impulse control. Records of histrionic patients, however, are generally much more benign in their content (reflecting a heavy reliance on defensive denial), whereas those of narcissistic patients often contain a high frequency of images of greatness and power.

Information derived from a Rorschach protocol enables a

clinical psychologist to assess an individual's total personality functioning, including his or her grasp of reality; defensive functioning; fears, wishes, and inner conflicts; symptomatology; affects; impulse control; and mental stability. The Rorschach test is generally used when an in-depth personality assessment is required or to assess personality functioning in individuals who are not responsive in clinical interview or to other, less labor-intensive methods.

Other projective measures along with the Rorschach test are often included in a personality assessment battery (Allison et al. 1968). Another well-known projective measure is the Thematic Apperception Test (TAT) (Bellack 1975; Tomkins 1947). The TAT consists of drawings of people in various attitudes. The patient is asked to make up a story for each picture. The degree of structure a test entails constitutes one of the major differences between it and projective measures. The TAT yields information analogous to that of the Rorschach test, translated into a reality-based (i.e., interpersonal) context. Because the TAT involves test stimuli that are much less ambiguous, it affords the patient greater opportunity to censor his or her responses. It is therefore important for an in-depth assessment of personality functioning to include measures that vary in their ambiguity. This enables the psychologist to assess the degree to which the patient depends on external structures to maintain his or her contact with reality.

Empirically Derived Tests

Empirically derived measures constitute the second major category of psychological tests used to assess personality functioning. The format for this type of test usually consists of a number of statements to which the patient answers "true" or "false." Test items are typically selected from a large pool of potential statements. Those items that best discriminate among patients in different diagnostic categories are retained, and this process is repeated until an adequate sample of items is selected. Only items that demonstrate empirical validity are retained, regardless of whether they reflect good "face validity." For example, answering "true" to item 181, "I do not have spells of hay fever or asthma," on the Minnesota Multiphasic Personality Inventory—2 (MMPI-2; Hathaway and McKinley 1989) clearly bears no relation to depressive symptomatology but is nevertheless scored on the MMPI-2 depression scale.

Personality assessment questionnaires have been widely used in clinical settings for the past 50 years. The best known (and still most widely used in North America) is the Minnesota Multiphasic Personality Inventory (MMPI) (Graham 1987; Hathaway and McKinley 1943; Lachar 1974; Marks and Seeman 1963). The MMPI was originally developed to assist in diagnosing various forms of mental illness. First published in 1942 (Hathaway and McKinley 1942) and most recently revised in 1989 (Hathaway and McKinley 1989), the MMPI currently consists of 567 items and yields scores on 3 validity scales, 10 clinical scales, 15 content scales, and 15 special scales (Butcher 1990; Butcher et al. 1989, 1990). Item content on the MMPI addresses a wide range of psychiatric symptoms, including suicidal ideation, obsessional thinking, manic states, paranoid ideation, anxiety states, depressive mood indicators, and schizophrenic thinking.

Of the two empirically derived personality assessment measures that are examined in this chapter and that are most widely used in clinical settings, the MMPI-2 requires the greater degree of inference. In interpreting the revised MMPI (the MMPI-2), all clinical scales elevated above 65 are combined into one-, two-, or three-point code types. Code types on the MMPI-2 have been shown to be associated with specific diagnostic categories, personality characteristics, and symptomatology. On the basis of code types (together with information derived from content scales), it is possible to generate hypotheses about a given patient's risk of committing suicide, defensive functioning, and general prognosis and to make treatment recommendations. Like the original version of the MMPI, the MMPI-2 demonstrates greater validity in the differential diagnosis of Axis I than Axis II disorders. Although the revised version of the MMPI was published several years after DSM-III (American Psychiatric Association 1980), it contains no scales specific to the differential diagnosis of Axis II disorders. The Morey Personality Disorder scales, derived from items on the original version of the MMPI (Morey et al. 1985, 1988), appeared to have potential utility for the differential diagnosis of DSM-III Axis II disorders. Recently, Colligan et al. (1994) published scale norms for the MMPI-2. (Seven of the Morey Personality Disorder scale items were omitted in the revised version of the MMPI.) However, to date there has been no research on the discriminant and predictive validity of the attenuated version of these scales with psychiatric patient populations.

The Millon Clinical Multiaxial Inventory (MCMI; Millon 1983) is a 175-item, true-false personality questionnaire. The revised MCMI (MCMI-II; Millon 1987) yields diagnoses on 13 personality disorder scales and contains a Validity Index and nine clinical syndrome scales. A score of greater than 74 on any of the MCMI-II personality disorder scales suggests a moderately severe level of personality dysfunction, whereas a score of greater than 85 generally indicates considerable impairment. In contrast with the MMPI-2, the format of the MCMI-II is congruent with that of DSM-III-R (American Psychiatric Association 1987).

Of the self-report inventories that can be used to diagnose specific personality disorders, only the MCMI has been widely used in clinical settings. Although extensive research on the original version of the MCMI has shown that it has low validity in the diagnosis of Axis I conditions (Patrick 1988), it possesses considerable utility in the differential diagnosis of personality disorders (Reich 1989). In the assignment of individual patient diagnoses, however, many of the personality disorder scales on the original MCMI showed only a moderate concordance with either clinicians' judgment or structured interviews (Cantrell and Dana 1987; Patrick 1993; Piersma 1987; Widiger et al. 1985). A recent study in which the original MCMI was compared with the MCMI-II (Inch and Crossley 1993) found that both versions overestimated the incidence of personality disorders in an outpatient psychiatric sample. Further research is needed to assess the discriminant and predictive validity of the MCMI-II personality disorder scales.

Before returning to the case example summarized at the beginning of this chapter, it is useful to gain a more complete understanding of the purposes served by the some of the personality assessment measures most frequently included in a test battery. In a brief psychological assessment, the MMPI-2 may be the only measure used and as such has a general diagnostic screening function with an emphasis on the diagnosis of Axis I pathology.

When empirically derived or objective measures of personality functioning are included in a test battery, they are generally administered and interpreted first, because their results are good indicators of what a patient is able and willing to disclose about himself or herself. In addition to the information they yield with regard to Axis I and Axis II pathology per se, these instruments can also suggest meaningful lines of inquiry to be pursued if a more in-depth assessment is required. Whenever more than one measure is administered, there must be an emphasis on integrating test data from all sources (as well as relevant background information and clinical observations). An outline and integration of the data obtained from both empirically derived (MMPI and MCMI) and projective measures (Rorschach and TAT) are illustrated in the following summary of Mr. A's test results:

> Mr. A was administered a test battery consisting of the MCMI, MMPI, Rorschach, and TAT. Valid profiles were generated on both the MMPI and the MCMI, and the results on the MMPI revealed significant contradictions. On the one hand, Mr. A sought to present himself in an improbably favorable light concerning his freedom from commonplace human frailties and exhibited a strong need to see himself (and to be seen by others) as an extremely virtuous person. Mr. A tended to somaticize his problems to a significant extent and to rely heavily on primitive denial. On the other hand, there were strong indications of profound identity confusion and impaired capacity for reality testing.
>
> On the MCMI, Mr. A reached threshold on the narcissistic personality disorder scale and was also found to have histrionic traits. Thus, he would be expected to have an inflated self-image and probably would be viewed by others as arrogant, with a general air of nonchalance, buoyant optimism, and cognitive expansiveness.
>
> On the Rorschach test, Mr. A's responses revealed considerable paranoia and mistrust (as expressed in his suspicions that he was being shown trick cards or that there were meaningful connections between the cards); also present were castration fears, sexual identity confusion, feared loss of control, autistic logic, and fears of being destroyed by malevolent forces. Mr. A's percepts on the Rorschach lacked plausibility and coherence. His efforts at integrating disparate elements of a given card were almost always unsuccessful. Some of his responses were perseverative (e.g., humans having the heads or features of animals were frequently seen).
>
> On the TAT, Mr. A's stories indicated that he was capable of

regaining reality contact in response to the greater degree of structure that this measure offers. His responses to the TAT pictures, however, were uniformly controlled, benign, and idealized (e.g., wrongdoers were forgiven and not punished, loud music was not played at parties, and everyone went home "at a decent hour").

Examination of Mr. A's test results from these four different measures allows us to become aware of the varying levels of his personality functioning. Specifically, test findings showed that Mr. A had been able to hide behind an acceptable social facade and had found ways of expressing his fears and unmet emotional needs that did not conflict with his positive self-image. Although this patient may be accurate in denying awareness of problems in any aspect of his daily life, his emotional equilibrium is actually very tenuous. It can readily be seen that Mr. A's pervasive striving for control, his inability to acknowledge any dissatisfaction with any aspect of his life, and his apparent self-confidence are all basically defensive in nature.

Test findings also showed that Mr. A is striving hard to keep out of conscious awareness his perceptions of the world as a threatening and chaotic place, his lack of a firm self-identity, and his image of himself as a helpless victim. We would not expect, therefore, that Mr. A's generalized anxiety symptoms and secondary dysphoria could be treated effectively by a direct, symptom-focused approach. Test findings show that Mr. A's presenting symptoms are serving the useful purpose of both containing and expressing the deeper sources of his distress and dysfunction. These findings dictate that a cautious, slow-paced, supportive approach to treatment would probably work best with this patient. It is probable that Mr. A sought professional help because at some level he had become aware that he lacked a firm grasp of reality and genuine self-acceptance and felt extremely vulnerable without knowing why. However, his pervasive mistrust of others and his justifiable fear of psychotic decompensation required that he not acknowledge these concerns. Treatment of this patient would therefore need to focus on the development of trust and, secondarily, on issues related to his self-identity.

The use of a battery of personality tests makes it possible to address Axis II pathology both categorically and dimensionally. The categorical approach to diagnosis refers to the use of discrete categories for the classification of personality disorders. This approach best conveys the uniqueness of individual patients when their test scores place them at the midpoint for a given diagnostic category. The dimensional approach to diagnosis refers to the classification of personality disorders along a continuum. This approach best conveys the uniqueness of individual patients whose test scores lie at the extremes of the score range for a given diagnostic category, as well as within the context of possible coexisting Axis I diagnoses.

As illustrated in the case example of Mr. A, results from a self-report measure of Axis I pathology (such as the MMPI-2) are initially examined to obtain an overview of the patient's symptom state, including the presence (or absence) of psychotic features, the degree of depression and anxiety, the level of available psychic energy, the degree of somatic concern, and the patient's willingness to respond in a nondefensive fashion. Next, results from objective measures of Axis II pathology (such as the MCMI-II) are examined for evidence of specific personality disorders or traits. Projective measures (the TAT and Rorschach) enable the clinician to understand the basic conflicts, wishes, and fears that underlie Mr. A's symptoms, attitudes, feelings, and behaviors and to recognize how these are expressed in his interpersonal relationships. Thus, in an in-depth assessment of personality functioning, data from empirically based and projective measures are combined and integrated to define salient aspects of an individual's personality with reference to specific referral questions.

Recently Developed Psychometric Measures of Personality Functioning

Research into the assessment of personality disorders during the past decade has led to the development of a number of dimensionally based instruments. Among these are the Neuroticism Extraversion Personality Inventory (NEO-PI; Costa and McCrae 1985), the Personality Assessment Inventory (PAI; Morey 1991), and the Tridimensional Personality Questionnaire (TPQ; Cloninger et al. 1991). Items on the revised version of the NEO-PI (NEO-PI-R) and the TPQ were selected on the basis of their capacity to capture an aspect of the dimensional typologies of personality on which each of these instruments is based. Unlike the MMPI-2 and the MCMI-II, these typologies do not specifically address either Axis I or Axis II pathology. The PAI, on the other hand, was designed to measure those clinical syndromes that in Morey's judgment encompassed the major categories of mental disorder and therefore is more congruent with DSM-III-R.

The NEO-PI was developed for use as a measure of Costa and McCrae's five-factor model of personality (Costa 1991; Costa and McCrae 1985, 1990, 1991, 1992; Miller 1991). In its most recent revision (1992), the NEO-PI-R includes two additional factors, "agreeableness" and "conscientiousness."

Research on the NEO-PI-R (and on preceding versions of this measure) has focused primarily on identifying personality traits in nonpsychiatric populations; most studies on this measure support Costa and McCrae's position that the NEO scales can identify the degree to which the personality traits specified are present. As Costa and McCrae indicate, the NEO-PI-R was not designed to diagnose pathology. However, they believe that this measure addresses some (if not all) dimensions of abnormal personality (as well as the major dimensions of normal personality) and have compiled a list of traits measured by the NEO-PI-R that they regard as related to each of the DSM-III-R personality disorders. They suggest that future research involving the administration of the NEO-PI-R to different diagnostic groups could establish prediction equations for the various scale scores. At this time, it would appear that the NEO-PI-R could best be used to enhance treatment strategies for patients with personality disorders by increasing the clinician's awareness of these individuals' basic "emotional, interpersonal, experiential, attitudinal, and motivational styles" (Costa and McCrae 1992, p. 346).

The PAI (Morey 1991) is an objective measure of psychopathology somewhat similar to the MMPI-2 in that it assesses a number of clinical syndromes. It also generates scale scores on borderline personality disorder traits, antisocial traits, substance abuse, aggression, suicidal ideation, perceived stress, perceived lack of support, responsivity to receiving treatment, dominance striving, and interpersonal warmth. Additionally, the PAI has four scales that assess response validity: inconsistency, infrequency, negative impression, and positive impression. The PAI potentially constitutes an improvement over the MMPI-2 in that it incorporates the concept of dimensionality (i.e., patients are asked to indicate the degree of endorsement for each item).

Research to date comparing patients' scores on PAI scales with scales (and subscales) on various other well-known measures of personality pathology (e.g., the MCMI-II, the MMPI-2, and the NEO-PI-R) suggest that the discriminant validity of this measure is potentially very good.

The TPQ was developed by Cloninger et al. (1991); it consists of 100 true-false items that address three interactive dimensions of personality: novelty seeking, harm avoidance, and reward dependence. Extreme scale scores on these three major subscales of the TPQ are identified with maladaptive personality functioning. The TPQ was developed to classify patients in accordance with Cloninger's eight categories of personality disorder; however, research to date on this correspondence has been quite limited. Some recent studies using this measure (Joffe et al. 1993; Wingerson et al. 1993) have demonstrated that the TPQ can successfully identify individuals within selected clinical populations who exhibit symptoms and/or behaviors consistent with TPQ constructs (e.g., patients who respond to antidepressant medication versus those who do not; those who comply with medication regimens versus noncompliant patients with anxiety disorders). Factor analytic studies, however, have yielded quite divergent findings.

At this point, the lack of research establishing the utility of the TPQ in the diagnosis and treatment of personality disorders argues against its independent use in clinical practice. The primary utility of the TPQ at this time would appear to lie in its capacity to generate meaningful prognostic statements with regard to patients who obtain scores showing specific patterns of personality traits. Such prognostic information can be extremely useful in treatment planning for individuals in particular patient populations (e.g., smokers). Although a number of other measures can serve this same purpose, recent research (Wetzel et al. 1992) has indicated that at least some aspects of personality functioning measured by the TPQ may not be addressed by more widely used personality assessment instruments, such as the MMPI-2. Thus, there seems to be sufficient evidence at this time to warrant the adjunctive, but not the independent, use of this instrument.

A number of non–empirically derived self-report measures specific to DSM-III-R Axis II pathology have also been developed over the last decade. The Personality Diagnostic Questionnaire (PDQ; Hyler et al. 1987), for example, is one measure on which there has been sufficient research with psychiatric populations to define its operating characteristics. To date it has not been widely used in clinical settings, although a software version has recently become commercially available that should increase its appeal to potential users.

In contrast to the other non–empirically derived measures mentioned, PDQ items represent a direct translation of every DSM-III-R criterion for each personality disorder. The revised version of the PDQ (the PDQ-R) consists of 152 items grouped according to each of the 11 DSM-III-R diagnostic categories; it also includes item sets for two provisional personality disorder categories (sadistic and self-defeating). An Impairment/Distress Index (designed to identify response bias) and two validity scales developed for the original version were also retained.

Research to date on the PDQ-R suggests that it tends to over-diagnose personality disorders (Hyler et al. 1990; Reich 1987). However, it also generates a very low rate of false-negative results; that is, clinicians can generally have a high degree of confidence that significant Axis II pathology is not present in patients who do not reach threshold on any of the PDQ-R scales. In addition, some PDQ-R scales may in fact be very appropriate for screening purposes. The PDQ-R Borderline Personality Disorder scale, for example, has been found to have good concordance with clinician-assigned diagnoses for individual patients (Hyler et al. 1989), and a better concordance than that obtained for the MCMI when the Structured Interview for the Diagnosis of Personality (Pfohl et al. 1985) was used as the criterion in assigning patients to this diagnostic category (Hyler et al. 1990). Given that the differential diagnosis of borderline personality disorder continues to be a primary concern for many treating clinicians in both inpatient and outpatient facilities, these findings, along with the extremely brief time required to complete and score the PDQ-R, recommend its wider use as a screening instrument.

The MMPI-2, the MCMI-II, the NEO-PI-R, the PAI, the PDQ-R, and the TPQ all possess the advantage of not being labor intensive; each can be administered individually or in a group format. Minimal time is required for administration and scoring of these questionnaires. Another significant advantage of these measures is that many patients are more willing to self-disclose when completing a self-report questionnaire than in a face-to-face interview.

Empirically derived measures such as the MMPI-2, the MCMI-II, the NEO-PI-R, the PAI, and the TPQ possess an additional advantage over most structured interview schedules in terms of their lower susceptibility to patients' efforts to censor their responses. Although no self-report measure can effectively guard against patients' ability to identify which items have an obviously pejorative connotation, most objective personality assessment measures (even those that are not empirically derived) include one or more scales that serve to indicate whether a patient has responded in a defensive or socially desirable fashion.

Although the MCMI-II probably constitutes the best currently available, empirically derived psychometric measure for the differential diagnosis of personality disorders, its independent use is generally contraindicated. It is much more likely to yield valid results when paired with the MMPI-2, because the latter measure is better adapted to identify coexistent Axis I pathology. Inclusion of the PDQ-R as well can assist in validating the existence of specific personality disorders identified by the MCMI-II; that is, the absence of any Axis II pathology on the PDQ-R would strongly suggest that any high scores obtained on MCMI-II syndrome scales probably reflect the impact of Axis I pathology on personality functioning.

The following case example illustrates how data from the MMPI, the MCMI, and the PDQ-R can be integrated in a brief assessment report to address the differential diagnosis and interactional aspects of Axis I and Axis II pathology.

Case 2

Mr. B, a 49-year-old married man, was referred to a specialty assessment team for evaluation of Axis II pathology. Mr. B had been unemployed for several years and had been recently admitted to a hospital for the treatment of bipolar affective disorder. Two different monoamine oxidase inhibitors had been tried, and he had had a series of six sessions of unilateral electroconvulsive therapy. He showed minimal improvement; his low frustration tolerance and concomitant threats of violence led to an early discharge under the care of his family doctor. Mr. B was referred to the assessment team by his family doctor because of the frequency of his office visits and his continuing threats of harming himself and others.

Mr. B generated valid results on the MMPI, the MCMI, and the PDQ-R. Test findings were most consistent with the following diagnoses:

- Axis I: dysthymic disorder, anxiety disorder
- Axis II: personality disorder not otherwise specified (avoidant, dependent, narcissistic, and paranoid features)

Test results showed Mr. B to be a fairly immature and egocentric individual who had little insight into his effect on others; his capacity or willingness to accept responsibility for his problems seemed to be very limited. He appeared to be trying to preserve his fragile self-esteem by projecting blame onto others and denying responsibility for his problems. Over time, however, reality supports for his defenses had clearly been eroded, and his dysphoria, suicidal ideation, and potential for self-harm had all greatly increased.

Test findings suggested that this patient tends to be vigilant and wary in his relationships with others; he anticipates rejection and seemingly has adopted a strategy of distancing and active withdrawing. However, Mr. B is not denying his longings for attention and affection; in fact, he makes a point of announcing that he is entitled to have these needs met and is alert to any evidence that his "rights" in this regard are being violated. This stance also serves to bolster his self-esteem and would probably be expressed either in his presenting himself as the victim of others' capriciousness and selfishness or, alternatively, in his seeking to have his needs met by intimidation and threats of violence. He would thus be able to feel powerful as well as self-righteous. For all his bluster, Mr. B is in fact a very passive and dependent individual. In that he is oversensitive to criticism, as well as fairly rigid and opinionated, others tend to experience his bids for reassurance, security, and guidance as burdensome.

Treatment Recommendations

Mr. B's potential for developing insight into his problems is very limited. In the context of a supportive relationship, however, he might be amenable to acquiring less abrasive ways of interacting with others. This type of patient tends to respond poorly to confrontation; he needs to experience confirmation of his perceptions (when possible) and validation of his self-worth.

It is not anticipated that this patient would show a particularly good response to anxiolytic and/or antidepressant medications, in that his Axis I symptoms are basically a manifestation of unmet narcissistic and dependency needs.

It may be noted that in both case examples presented, there was evidence of more than one type of Axis I and Axis II pathology (comorbidity).[1] When a patient's test record shows significant evidence of specific traits of one or more personality disorders, a diagnosis of personality disorder not otherwise specified is generally assigned.

Stability of Psychometric Assessment of Personality Disorders

Clinicians and diagnosticians recognize that personality (and personality pathology) involves highly complex concepts that may be viewed in a multiplicity of ways. Given the goal of understanding personality disorders in ways that are clinically useful, that is, in ways that allow findings to be readily translated into therapeutic strategies, it is important to bear in mind that the stability of any assessment approach is only relative. Although the clinical status of patients is automatically updated and reevaluated each time they are interviewed, the fact that it is just as essential to periodically obtain an update of personality assessment results is easily overlooked. Although by definition personality disorders constitute chronic, long-standing, dysfunctional patterns of behavior, to some degree all assessment findings reflect the impact of transient state variables. Although projective test results are not as readily vulnerable to erosion, over the course of time (particularly with the occurrence of significant positive and/or negative life events), changes in personality structure and functioning can occur, and these are typically reflected in both empirically derived and projective test findings. It is well known,

---

[1] *Comorbidity* refers to the fact that patients' test scores may meet the criteria for more than one Axis I or Axis II disorder. To date, prescriptive therapies for patients diagnosed as comorbid for two or more disorders have not been well defined, although generally Axis I pathology is assigned a higher treatment priority.

for example, that results obtained on personality assessment measures during the course of a psychiatric hospitalization often show significantly more pathology than when the same measures are repeated after discharge.

It is therefore important, when test results are used to assist in therapeutic management, to take into consideration the patient's personal circumstances at the time of assessment and to give serious consideration to repeating personality testing when major changes occur or at an interval of no longer than 1 year after the original assessment was completed. Updating personality assessment results will not only lead to a more valid ongoing utilization of test findings but will also help to determine whether the treatment approach currently being used with a given patient is having any impact on those aspects of personality pathology judged to be most problematic.

Overview of Computer-Generated Reports for the MMPI-2 and MCMI-II

Computer-generated reports that are now available for both the MMPI-2 and the MCMI-II are quite extensively used. A number of scoring and interpretive services market computer scoring and/or report programs, personality profiles, or narrative reports for both the MMPI-2 and MCMI-II. The cost of these services varies according to volume and service provider, but in virtually all instances a computer-generated report is less expensive to purchase than one that is clinician generated. The inexperienced consumer, however, would do well to heed certain caveats.

First, examine how computerized MMPI reports are generated. After test data for a specific patient are entered into the computer, they are transformed into numerical scores on each of the various MMPI-2 scales. The narrative program selects all interpretive statements that conform to single-scale and profile configuration scores for each set of individual patient data entered. These statements are printed out in a narrative format; to a limited extent, the narrative can be further refined by including basic demographic data on each patient.

One important constraint on the quality and accuracy of computer-generated interpretive statements or narrative reports is that there is only limited provision for the inclusion of relevant data gathered from the patient's personal history or from the interview. In many respects, computer-generated reports are little better than "blind" interpretations of the test data.

Most psychologists now use computer software programs for scoring tests such as the MMPI-2 and MCMI-II; computer-generated interpretive statements may also be used, with a view to saving time and effort. No existing report service, however, has succeeded in eliminating the need for a psychologist to select which narrative statements are really consistent with a specific patient's clinical presentation and history. If all statements included in an interpretive program have been selected "actuarially," they can be said to accurately describe or predict behaviors, symptoms, or attitudes common to most of the individuals who obtain scores within a given scale range or who obtain a particular score pattern. Of necessity, such reports will contain more generalities than will clinician-generated reports, which can integrate all relevant patient information. Most computer-generated narratives, however, do not consist exclusively of empirically derived interpretive statements; thus, their usefulness also hinges on the knowledge and experience of the clinician who developed the particular interpretive program. As Graham (1990) stated, adequate validity has not yet been established for any of the computer-generated MMPI-2 narrative reports currently available.

A slightly different situation prevails for the MCMI-II. To date, computer-generated MCMI profiles and narrative reports have been made commercially available only through National Computer Services. According to Millon (1987), the major portion of the descriptor statements that constitute the MCMI-II narratives are derived from actuarial data; the remainder have been derived from Millon's own theory of personality functioning (Millon 1981).

The Referral Process

Information-sharing constitutes the essence of the referral process. The degree to which a psychological assessment can meet the needs of the referring clinician rests heavily on the clinician's success in communicating the purpose of the referral to the patient and eliciting his or her cooperation. It is not unusual for patients to view a referral for personality assessment as threatening or intrusive. These reactions are almost always intensified by the presence of Axis II pathology and lead to evasive responding, denial of problems and symptoms, and poor motivation. In addition to offering an explanation for the referral, the referring clinician should make every effort to assist the patient who manifests symptoms of personality dysfunction to view the referral and the assessment as a collaborative effort. The potential benefits of the referral should be stated as explicitly as possible (e.g., that the information contained in the assessment report is likely to enhance the clinician's efforts to help the patient and will provide information that will be useful to the patient in terms of his or her self-understanding, self-management, and decision making).

The clinical psychologist to whom the patient is referred also requires more than minimal identifying information in order to thoroughly and precisely address the referral question(s). The following guidelines indicate the kind of information that is most useful to include in making a referral for personality assessment:

- A summary of the patient's medical, social, and vocational history
- A description of the patient's current functioning and presenting problems
- A summary of observational and other data that have led to the consideration of a diagnosis of personality disorder
- An outline of specific issues or questions that the referring clinician wishes to see addressed

Ideally, the clinician's referral question will serve a central organizing function for the assessment. Too often, however, referring clinicians neglect to mention the specific issues they wish to have addressed. There are various reasons for this omission. Some clinicians may fear that specific referral questions will narrow the scope of inquiry and that important information will be missed; others do not wish to bias the data interpretation and therefore also prefer to provide only minimal background information. Psychiatrists and general practitioners, who are more accustomed to ordering laboratory investigations, might not hesitate to specify the specific psychometric instruments to be used (an unnecessary and undesirable constraint), while failing to appreciate how much their own hypotheses, observations, background information, and specific questions can contribute to the ultimate utility of the assessment report.

Conclusion

Psychometric assessment measures can offer most assistance to the clinician when they are used to maximize knowledge of the patient with a personality disorder as an individual. Although categorical approaches to the classification of personality dysfunction (e.g., DSM-IV [American Psychiatric Association 1994] Axis II diagnoses) can yield a good descriptive picture of patients' most prominent symptoms and personality traits, they are much less comprehensive than dimensional approaches, which assess patients on various aspects of personality functioning.

Accuracy in the diagnosis of personality disorders per se is most efficiently achieved by the judicious selection and combination of standardized psychometric assessment measures, chosen to accord with the specific referral question(s). In most cases this would entail addressing the issue of comorbidity (assessment of Axis I pathology) by using an empirically derived measure such as the MMPI-2, together with one or more self-report measures of Axis II pathology. In clinical practice, recognition of the merits of dimensional assessment of personality dysfunction will increasingly be reflected in the inclusion of dimensionally structured Axis II self-report measures in the psychological test battery.

Most approaches to the assessment of personality disorders depend on either the skills of an external observer or the patient's own conscious awareness for the accurate delineation of traits, symptoms, and behaviors. As a result, even the increasingly popular dimensional approaches to assessment are limited to locating a patient along a continuum consisting of points established between the extremes for various personality traits. Although dimensional approaches offer significant advantages over categorical diagnostic systems, they remain essentially descriptive measures. Neither categorical nor dimensional approaches constitute interactive approaches to personality assessment, because they leave untapped the information not available to the patient's conscious awareness, and they fail to elucidate the relationship (represented by symptoms and maladaptive behaviors) that the patient has established between his or her inner and outer worlds.

Typically in clinical practice, a categorical diagnosis, together with a description of symptoms and/or a dimensional presentation of personality traits, is either sufficient or all that it is feasible to obtain. However, in instances when this level of understanding proves inadequate for the purpose of developing an effective treatment approach, it becomes necessary to gain access to the wealth of clinical data that lies beyond the barrier imposed by the patient's conscious awareness and his or her desire and capacity for self-disclosure. This task is best approached through the use of projective techniques. Projective techniques are not very frequently used because they are labor intensive and require extensive experience and training on the part of the examiner; hence their potential value is often ignored. It is not suggested that categorically and dimensionally based psychometric measures be set aside in favor of projective techniques. As the case examples in this chapter indicate, the use of these measures in clinical practice would in almost all instances complement one another.

With access to the multiplicity of approaches to the assessment of personality functioning afforded by psychometric techniques, the treating clinician can move far beyond the level of differential diagnosis of personality disorders and/or treatment limited to efforts at symptom reduction or containment of maladaptive behaviors. As the case examples in this chapter illustrate, the various psychometrically based techniques available for the assessment of personality disorders can provide considerable assistance to the treating clinician in avoiding the therapeutic and management failures that have tended to be endemic to this patient population.

References

Allison J, Blatt S, Zimit C: The Interpretation of Psychological Tests. New York, Harper & Row, 1968

American Psychiatric Association: Diagnostic and Statistical Manual of Mental Disorders, 3rd Edition. Washington, DC, American Psychiatric Association, 1980

American Psychiatric Association: Diagnostic and Statistical Manual of Mental Disorders, 3rd Edition, Revised. Washington, DC, American Psychiatric Association, 1987

American Psychiatric Association: Diagnostic and Statistical Manual of Mental Disorders, 4th Edition. Washington, DC, American Psychiatric Association, 1994

Anastasi A: Psychological Testing, 6th Edition. New York, Macmillan, 1988

Aronow E, Reznikoff M: Rorschach Content Interpretation. New York, Grune & Stratton, 1976

Bellack L: The TAT, CAT, and SAT in Clinical Use. New York, Grune & Stratton, 1975

Butcher J: Assessing Patients in Psychotherapy: Use of the MMPI-2 for Treatment Planning. New York, Oxford University Press, 1990

Butcher J, Dahlstrom W, Graham J, et al: Minnesota Multiphasic Personality Inventory (MMPI-2). Manual for Administration and Scoring. Minneapolis, University of Minnesota Press, 1989

Butcher J, Graham J, Williams C, et al: Development and Use of the MMPI-2 Content Scales. Minneapolis, University of Minnesota Press, 1990

Cantrell J, Dana R: Use of the Millon Clinical Multiaxial Inventory (MCMI) as a screening instrument at a community mental health center. J Clin Psychol 43:366–375, 1987

Cloninger CR, Przybeck TR, Svrakic DM: The Tridimensional Personality Questionnaire: US normative data. Psychol Rep 69:1047–1057, 1991

Colligan RC, Morey LC, Offord KP: The MMPI/MMPI-2 Personality Disorder scales: contemporary norms for adults and adolescents. J Clin Psychol 50:168–199, 1994

Costa PT: Clinical use of the five-factor model: an introduction. J Pers Assess 57:393–398, 1991

Costa PT, McCrae RR: The NEO Personality Inventory Manual. Odessa, FL, Psychological Assessment Resources, 1985

Costa PT, McCrae RR: Personality disorders and the five-factor model of personality. Journal of Personality Disorders 4:362–371, 1990

Costa PT, McCrae RR: The Revised NEO-PI-R Inventory Manual. Odessa, FL, Psychological Assessment Resources, 1991

Costa PT, McCrae RR: The five-factor model of personality and its relevance to personality disorders. Journal of Personality Disorders 6:343–359, 1992

Graham J: The MMPI: A Practical Guide, 2nd Edition. New York, Oxford University Press, 1987

Graham J: The MMPI-2: Assessing Personality and Psychopathology. New York, Oxford University Press, 1990

Hathaway S, McKinley J: A multiphasic personality schedule: the measurement of symptomatic depression. J Psychol 14:73–84, 1942

Hathaway S, McKinley J: Minnesota Multiphasic Personality Inventory. Minneapolis, University of Minnesota, 1943

Hathaway S, McKinley J: Minnesota Multiphasic Personality Inventory—2. Minneapolis, University of Minnesota, 1989

Hirschfeld R: Personality disorders: definition and diagnosis. Journal of Personality Disorders 7 (suppl):9–17, 1993

Hyler S, Reider R, Williams J, et al: The Personality Diagnostic Questionnaire—Revised (PDQ-R). New York, New York State Psychiatric Institute, Biometrics Research, 1987

Hyler S, Reider R, Williams J, et al: A comparison of clinical and self-report diagnoses of DSM-III personality disorders in 552 patients. Compr Psychiatry 30:170–178, 1989

Hyler S, Skodol A, Kellman H, et al: Validity of the Personality Diagnostic Questionnaire—Revised: comparison with two structured interviews. Am J Psychiatry 147:1043–1048, 1990

Inch R, Crossley D: Diagnostic utility of the MCMI-I and MCMI-II with psychiatric outpatients. J Clin Psychol 49:358–366, 1993

Joffe RT, Bagby RM, Levitt AJ, et al: The Tridimensional Personality Questionnaire in major depression. Am J Psychiatry 150:959–960, 1993

Kwawer J, Lerner H, Lerner P, et al: Borderline Phenomenon and the Rorschach Test. New York, International Universities Press, 1980

Lachar D: The MMPI: Clinical Assessment and Automated Interpretations. Los Angeles, CA, Western Psychological Services, 1974

Marks P, Seeman W: The Actuarial Description of Abnormal Personality: An Atlas for Use with the MMPI. Baltimore, MD, Williams & Wilkins, 1963

Miller T: The psychotherapeutic utility of the five-factor model of personality: a clinician's experience. J Pers Assess 57:449–464, 1991

Millon T: Disorders of Personality: DSM-III, Axis II. New York, Wiley Interscience, 1981

Millon T: Millon Clinical Multiaxial Inventory Manual, 3rd Edition. Minneapolis, MN, National Computer Systems, 1983

Millon T: Manual for the MCMI-II, 2nd Edition. Minneapolis, MN, National Computer Systems, 1987

Morey L: Personality Assessment Inventory. Odessa, FL, Psychological Assessment Resources, 1991

Morey L, Waugh M, Blashfield R: MMPI scales for DSM-III personality disorders: their derivation and correlates. J Pers Assess 49:245–251, 1985

Morey L, Blashfield R, Webb W, et al: MMPI scales for DSM-III personality disorders: a preliminary validation study. J Clin Psychol 44:47–50, 1988

Patrick J: Concordance of the MCMI and the MMPI in the diagnosis of three DSM-III Axis I disorders. J Clin Psychol 44:186–190, 1988

Patrick J: Validation of the MCMI-I Borderline Personality Disorder scale with a well-defined criterion sample. J Clin Psychol 49:28–32, 1993

Pfohl B, Stangl D, Zimmerman M: A structured interview for the DSM-III personality disorders: a preliminary report. Arch Gen Psychiatry 42:591–596, 1985

Piersma H: The MCMI as a measure of DSM-III Axis II diagnoses: an empirical comparison. J Clin Psychol 43:478–483, 1987

Rabin A: Projective Techniques in Personality Assessment. New York, Springer, 1968

Rapaport D, Gill M, Schafer R: Diagnostic Psychological Testing. Chicago, IL, Year Book Medical, 1945

Reich J: Instruments measuring DSM-III and DSM-III-R personality disorders. Journal of Personality Disorders 1:220–240, 1987

Reich J: Update on instruments to measure DSM-III and DSM-III-R personality disorders. J Nerv Ment Dis 177:366–370, 1989

Schafer R: Clinical Application of Psychological Tests. New York, International Universities Press, 1954

Singer M: Borderline diagnosis and psychological tests, in Borderline Personality Disorders. Edited by Hartcollis P. New York, International Universities Press, 1977, pp 193–212

Tomkins S: Thematic Apperception Test. New York, Grune & Stratton, 1947

Wetzel R, Knesevich M, Brown S, et al: Correlates of Tridimensional Personality Questionnaire scales with selected Minnesota Multiphasic Personality Inventory scales. Psychol Rep 71:1027–1038, 1992

Widiger T, Williams J, Spitzer R, et al: The MCMI as a measure of DSM-III. J Pers Assess 49:366–383, 1985

Wingerson D, Sullivan M, Dager S, et al: Personality traits and early discontinuation from clinical trials in anxious patients. J Clin Psychopharmacol 13:194–197, 1993

CHAPTER 4

Neuropsychiatric Issues in the Management of Personality Disorders

Robert van Reekum, M.D., F.R.C.P.C.

*I*t is possible that many of the readers of this book on personality disorders will be surprised to see a chapter devoted to neuropsychiatric issues in the management of personality disorders. Indeed, most of the twentieth-century literature related to personality in general and, consequently, to disordered personalities is to be found in the psychoanalytic literature. Thus, most of our conceptions about personality are devoid of considerations relating to the involvement of the mind's biological substrate, the brain. More recently, however, empirical research has begun to reveal the importance of an intact brain in the formation and maintenance of normal personality.

In this chapter, I very briefly review the evidence relating to brain involvement in personality disorders. Interested readers are referred to more complete reviews. I then provide a case illustration. Neuropsychiatric methods of assessment are provided and are targeted to the non-neuropsychiatrist. The chapter concludes with a review of treatment options derived from these considerations. The text is summarized in Table 4–1.

Table 4–1.   Summary

Assessment

1. Neurodevelopmental history—careful inquiry into developmental or acquired brain lesions

2. Neurodevelopmental syndrome inventories—characteristic phenomena seen after brain injuries (e.g., adult attention-deficit hyperactivity disorder, seizures)

3. A full neurological examination, including a metabolic workup

4. Neurological soft sign assessment

5. Neurological investigations (e.g., electroencephalography, brain mapping, positron-emission tomography)

6. Neurocognitive testing

Treatment

1. Pharmacological management of underlying neurobehavioral disorder(s)

2. Cognitive-behavioral rehabilitation

3. Modification of existing therapies based on identified deficits

4. Increased understanding of and improved caring for patients with personality disorders through psychoeducation

The Brain and Personality: Brief Review of the Evidence

Elliott (1986) nicely summarized the historical evolution of our understanding of the role of the brain in forming the personality. In addition, he cites evidence from genetic, neurological soft-sign, electroencephalogram (EEG), and neurocognitive studies to establish the underlying role of the brain in persons with antisocial personality disorder. The family history studies show that persons with antisocial personality disorder and alcoholic patients derive from a "common genetic pool" (Elliott 1986, p. 230). Persistent excessive bilateral theta activity is seen in the EEGs of patients with aggressive antisocial personality disorder. Cognitive testing suggests brain dysfunction, as do abnormal psychogalvanic responses and resistance to the establishment of conditioned reflexes.

Research on the involvement of the brain in other personality disorders is in a very early stage. Weintraub and Mesulam (1983) studied 14 subjects with early-onset, persistent "shyness" and found evidence of right-hemisphere brain damage. These subjects did not receive a formal psychiatric assessment. The case descriptions, however, suggest that a number of these subjects had avoidant personality disorder. The investigators suggest that these persons have a form of dyslexia, or learning disability, that specifically involves the right hemisphere and thus affects nonverbal interpersonal skills and emotional stability.

I review the case for the involvement of the brain in causing borderline personality disorder elsewhere (van Reekum 1993). There is a reasonably strong association between borderline personality disorder and a history of developmental or acquired brain injury. Developmental diagnoses frequently include attention-deficit hyperactivity disorder (ADHD), learning disabilities, developmental delays (e.g., persistent enuresis), and perinatal events. Acquired diagnoses frequently include traumatic brain injury, seizures, and other central nervous system insults (e.g., anoxia, encephalitis).

Subjects with borderline personality disorder have also been studied prospectively. EEG abnormalities are frequently found, whereas computed tomography (CT) abnormalities are rare. At least two neurological soft signs (further discussed later in this chapter) are found in 60% or more of patients with borderline personality disorder.

The presence of soft signs seems to distinguish patients with borderline personality disorder from control subjects without borderline personality disorder and from depressed control subjects. Cognitive testing of language, memory, and visuospatial and motor functioning has revealed few difficulties in these realms in subjects with borderline personality disorder. Testing of frontal system functioning, however, appears to reveal deficits, most notably impulsivity, cognitive inflexibility, and poor self-monitoring, sequencing, perseveration, and information processing. These deficits may well contribute to the behavioral, interpersonal, and emotional difficulties exhibited by patients with borderline personality disorder and furthermore may have a significant impact on psychotherapeutic efforts. For example, frontal system dysfunction will make it harder for subjects with borderline personality disorder to put into practice the gains they have made in therapy. The often-quoted observation that subjects with borderline personality disorder seem to learn in session and then fail out of session may thus have an identifiable cognitive basis. Later in this chapter, I review tests that can demonstrate these deficits and make some suggestions for modifications to psychotherapy that may result in greater treatment gains.

The role of neurotransmitters, hormonal functioning, and neuropeptides in producing altered behavior or personality is beyond the scope of this chapter. Interested readers are referred to other sources (Coccaro et al. 1989; Gardner et al. 1990). Reviews related to pharmacological manipulation of these systems also exist (Soloff et al. 1986; see also Chapter 6). I limit my discussion of pharmacological interventions to those that are of relevance to underlying brain pathology, and perhaps, therefore, can be expected to have a secondary impact on personality disorder symptoms and behaviors (see "Treatment Implications" section below).

In summary, there is increasing evidence for a role of the brain in determining personality functioning. Developmental right-hemisphere dysfunction may contribute to avoidant personality disorder, frontal system impairment to borderline personality disorder, and widespread cortical dysfunction to antisocial personality disorder. The behavioral similarities between patients with schizoid personality disorder and those with the negative symptoms of schizophrenia point to possible involvement of the dorsolateral prefrontal cortex in schizoid personality disorder. Patients with schizotypal and paranoid personality disorder may have dysfunction in limbic or limbic striatum (i.e., anterior basal ganglia) areas.

Although it is clear that much more research is required, for the clinician these considerations hold the promise of future effective biological and cognitive/behavioral treatments and indicate the need for a thorough neurodevelopmental history and examination. Given the lack of strong research evidence to date, treatment interventions initiated as the result of these assessments will need to be closely evaluated on an individual basis. Single-subject, randomized, placebo-controlled trials, or N of 1 studies, are described herein as a potentially useful method for ensuring nonbiased, systematic evaluation of drug efficacy and side effects (Guyatt et al. 1988).

Neuropsychiatric Assessment

Six aspects of the assessment are considered here: neurodevelopmental history, neurobehavioral syndrome inventories, the neurological examination, the neurological soft-sign examination, neurological investigations, and neurocognitive testing.

Neurodevelopmental History

Full descriptions of neurodevelopmental histories can be found in standard neurology and psychiatry texts. A brief screening history is described here. A history of in utero and perinatal injuries can be explored by asking about the mother's health during pregnancy. Was there evidence of drugs, alcohol, medications, or smoking during pregnancy? Was the pregnancy full term or preterm? Was there a normal birth weight? Was the patient a "blue baby" (i.e., one with a low Apgar score)? Was there a lengthy hospital stay after birth or a need for readmission, neonatal intensive care, or incubator? Clearly, an interview with a parent, supplemented by hospital records, will assist with the developmental history; however, reasonably good data are often available from the patient when probed in this focused manner.

Reliably reported developmental milestones include walking by age 12–18 months, single spoken words by 12 months, and bowel and bladder control by age 4–5 years. Few older patients have had formal assessments for learning disabilities, but younger patients may well have had learning or psychological assessments at school or through their family physician. Some may even have been given a formal diagnosis of dyslexia or learning disability. For those who have not been formally assessed, a history of trouble with spelling, reading, or arithmetic in the early school years can point to a possible learning disability. The presumptive diagnosis is strengthened by a history of normal learning in other areas (ruling out the likelihood of mental retardation) and by a history of remedial schoolwork or special education.

Childhood diagnoses of ADHD were often made in the past, and typically patients will recall being told they were "hyperactive" or needed "something to slow me down" (e.g., methylphenidate [Ritalin]). For those that did not receive a formal assessment or diagnosis, a retrospective assessment of ADHD symptoms can be attempted (ideally supplemented by second-person histories or school reports). However, the retrospective assessment done with adults may fail to demonstrate all of the necessary symptoms. To improve diagnostic confidence, a neurobehavioral symptom inventory has been developed to assess persistent/adult symptoms of ADHD. These symptoms seem to be present in a sizable minority of all adults who had childhood ADHD. This inventory is presented later in this chapter.

The neurodevelopmental history for acquired brain injuries is similar to the traditional neurological history. Special attention should be paid to emotional and behavioral changes occurring in the months and years following such injuries. I specifically inquire into episodes of head trauma and ask questions about loss of consciousness and its duration; the need for hospitalization; and any immediate sequelae, such as poor attention, arousal, or memory, and headaches, irritability, or poor judgment. Did the patient require any neurosurgical or pharmacological interventions? Did he or she receive EEG, CT or magnetic resonance imaging (MRI) scans, or neuropsychological (cognitive) testing? In regard to other acquired neurological events, a question such as "Have you ever had a neurological disease?" is rarely productive. This kind of general inquiry should be followed up by specific questions about structural birth defects, polio, syphilis, cerebral palsy, chromosomal abnormalities, meningitis, encephalitis (or "brain infections"), and Parkinson's disease. A similarly thorough family neurological history is essential. In gathering information about seizures, the examiner needs to remember that generalized, tonic-clonic seizures represent only a fraction of all seizure types. A neurobehavioral inventory to assess patients for simple or complex partial seizures is included in the following section.

Neurobehavioral Syndrome Inventories

The book *Clinical Neuropsychiatry* by Cummings (1985) is an excellent source for expected symptoms and signs of neurobehavioral disorders. When assessing for simple or complex partial seizures, the following experiential domains can be considered to provide a structure to the history:

- *Sensory phenomena* are visual, olfactory, gustatory, or tactile hallucinations. Auditory hallucinations may also occur but are less specific, also occurring in disorders such as schizophrenia. Illusions (or sensory distortions) may also occur.

- *Affective phenomena* may be any emotion, most commonly fear and anger.
- *Motor phenomena* may involve any muscle group, usually repetitive jerks or tremorlike movements, but may also involve highly complex motor programs. These sometimes progress to other muscle groups (as is seen in jacksonian epilepsy).
- *Cognitive symptomatology* consists of feelings of déjà vu (the mental impression that a new experience has happened before), jamais vu (feeling that a familiar environment is foreign), dissociative experiences, repetitive or intrusive thoughts or memories, and alterations in one's sense of time.
- *Impairment of consciousness* is a feature that distinguishes complex from simple partial seizures.

Many of these phenomena are nonspecific, difficult to elucidate, and often difficult to interpret. The following features will heighten the index of suspicion that these phenomena are indeed related to seizure activity:

- Rapid onset
- Context independent (do not occur exclusively in particular situations; e.g., fear occurring only in crowded places is more suggestive of panic attacks or agoraphobia)
- Occur while the patient is asleep
- Typically highly repetitive ("I always see the same thing")
- Usually brief (lasting a few minutes typically; longer durations do not exclude the diagnosis of seizures and probably represent status epilepticus occurring focally)
- Postictal period of drowsiness, confusion, or mood change

Although an EEG can assist with the diagnosis of seizures, EEGs are insensitive, especially for seizure foci buried deep within the limbic system. The correct interpretation of a negative EEG is not that the patient does not have seizures but rather that the EEG did not give further evidence of seizures. The sensitivity of the EEG can be improved by sleep deprivation and through the use of more invasive electrode placement. Ultimately, however, the diagnosis may remain in question until a treatment trial has been undertaken. Careful monitoring of event frequency and severity and duration both before and during the trial is essential and may be aided by the use of N of 1 designs.

Wender et al. (1985) developed an instrument to assess ADHD symptoms persisting into adulthood. During screening, clinicians may ask the patient whether he or she has

1. Persistent motor hyperactivity (e.g., restlessness, difficulty relaxing, being "always on the go," feelings of sadness or discomfort when inactive)?
2. Persistent attention deficits (e.g., trouble concentrating on conversation or reading, frequent forgetfulness)?
   If the answer to both of these questions is "no," stop here. If either or both answers are "yes," proceed to:
3. Rapid and brief (over hours or days) changes in mood?
4. Difficulty completing tasks (poorly organized, change tasks before their completion)?
5. Impulsivity (frequent changes in jobs or relationships, shopping sprees with consequent financial difficulties, reckless driving)?
6. Stress intolerance (react strongly to stress with anxiety, depression, confusion, or anger, leading to repeated crises)?
7. Inability to maintain relationships over time?

It should be noted that Wender et al. require that a childhood diagnosis of ADHD be present before the adult diagnosis is made and that the above symptoms be long-standing. Other neurobehavioral sequelae (such as interictal personality changes and postconcussion symptoms) can be found in Cummings' text (1985) and other textbooks of neuropsychiatry.

Neurological Examination

I do not review the neurological examination herein but rather emphasize the need for a careful neurological examination in all psychiatrically impaired persons. In addition, a careful functional inquiry and metabolic workup may reveal contributory systemic illnesses.

Neurological Soft Signs

The term *soft* is unfortunate in that it may be understood that neurological soft signs are only weakly predictive of brain dysfunction. This is not the case. Rather, the term is meant to signify the inability of such signs to localize brain dysfunction. The presence of a number of soft signs can contribute to one's confidence in diagnosing brain pathology. Examples of such signs include the following:

- *Sequential finger-thumb opposition*—The examiner should observe for evidence of "overflow movements," in which the inactive hand begins to mirror the active hand; dystonias in either hand; and gross asymmetries in performance.
- *Tandem gait*—This sign is characterized by heel-to-toe walking; the examiner should also note arm or hand dystonias.
- *Stress gait*—The examiner should ask the patient to walk on the lateral edge of his or her feet, noting arm or hand dystonias.
- *Rhythmic foot-tapping*—The examiner should note arrhythmias.
- *Alternating sequence completion*—The examinee should continue the following patterns:
  m n m n m n
  or alternating squares and triangles, while the examiner notes perseverations.
- *Luria three-step (fist-palm-side test)*—The examiner demonstrates these sequential hand movements and observes the examinee's ability to complete the task repetitively. Inability to succeed, especially when given verbal cues, indicates brain (especially frontal system) involvement.

Neurological Investigations

CT and MRI scans appear to be indicated only when a history of structural brain damage (such as that which may occur with tumors or severe traumatic brain injuries) is suspected. EEGs may well be helpful. The presence of spike and wave activity is diagnostic for seizures. Nonspecific widespread EEG abnormalities are commonly found in patients with antisocial personality disorder and borderline personality disorder, again raising the suspicion of underlying brain involvement. Quantified EEG techniques (i.e., brain mappings) may be of promise in the future.

Similarly, other techniques to study brain function, such as positron-emission tomography, may also play a role. The research to date, using techniques in probands with personality disorders, is sparse.

Neurocognitive Testing

Several structured neurocognitive screening examinations are available. A word of caution, however: Many of these examinations have been tested for use in severely impaired subjects, such as institutionalized patients with dementia, and their sensitivity and validity in other populations is therefore suspect. I have found the Neurobehavioral Cognitive Screening Examination (Schwamm et al. 1987) to be reasonably sensitive in subjects with traumatic brain injury (clinical observation only). With any screening examination, however, perfect scores do not rule out underlying brain pathology; a full neuropsychological assessment may be needed to fully understand and appreciate subtle cognitive difficulties. Other sources of screening neurocognitive examinations include the works of Cummings (1985) and Mesulam (1985).

A thorough neuropsychological assessment will include much more than an IQ test and measures of "posterior," or basic, functioning such as language, memory, and visuospatial spheres. Careful attention to the many aspects of arousal and attention, psychomotoric speed, and frontal system functioning are also essential. The reader of neuropsychological reports should be careful to look for terms such as *abstractional abilities, mental/cognitive flexibility, insight, sequencing and planning abilities, ability to receive and adapt to feedback, fluency,* and *evidence of impulsivity and/or perseveration.*

Difficulties in these higher-order cognitive tasks provide evidence of frontal system dysfunction.

Treatment Implications

Pharmacological

Occasionally, pharmacological interventions are suggested by the finding of a possibly causative underlying neurobehavioral disorder. Two examples are provided by the use of methylphenidate in patients with persistent ADHD (Hooberman and Stern 1984) and carbamazepine in patients with seizure disorders (Cowdry and Gardner 1988). As in the case example provided, the need for careful monitoring of cognitive, behavioral, and affective outcomes is essential. This process can be facilitated by the N of 1 study methodology (Guyatt et al. 1988).

Rehabilitative

Cognitive rehabilitation may increase the ability to receive, integrate, and utilize new learning. Secondary symptomatic relief from personality disorders and associated anxiety and affective disorders may result. Improved responses to psychotherapy may also be seen. Cognitive therapy generally has been shown to be effective in improving cognitive function, although more study is required (Diller and Gordon 1981; Levin 1990; Volpe and McDowell 1990). It appears that some cognitive abilities are more amenable to change than others, and the specific deficits associated with personality disorders have yet to be defined. Finally, the ability of cognitive therapy to have a secondary impact on mood, anxiety, and personality disorder traits has not been shown.

Cognitive rehabilitation will not always be available. In these cases, other treatment implications will still apply (see "Modification of Existing Psychotherapeutic Modalities" and "Recognition of Patients' Deficits" later in this chapter). In addition, the therapist may take on a problem-solving or teaching role with an eye not toward "curing" the deficits but rather toward devising ways in which the patient and his or her family and environment may adapt to these deficits, thus enhancing the patient's functioning. Such adaptations may be as relatively simple as the use of a memory book for patients with memory disorders or as complex as the use of family members to act as "surrogate frontal lobes" by assisting with self-monitoring, problem solving, and other tasks.

Behavioral rehabilitation strategies are widely used in brain-injured populations (Burke and Lewis 1986; Hollon 1973; Wood 1987), and Linehan (1989) has proposed a related methodology for use in treating impulsive or suicidal borderline personality disorder patients. Where available, expertise with these techniques should be sought, but such services will be difficult to find and, often, to fund. The treating therapist may borrow some general principles from these techniques, however, and therefore further reading and learning about behavior rehabilitation is to be encouraged in all persons working with patients with personality disorders. I favor behavioral strategies emphasizing the positive reinforcement of adaptive behaviors over those that focus on the extinction of maladaptive behaviors. Reinforcement techniques are multiple; the token economy and the use of social praise and displeasure are two such techniques.

Modified Psychotherapeutic Modalities

Modifying existing psychotherapeutic modalities on the basis of identified cognitive deficits may improve psychotherapy outcomes. Motivation, insight, and the ability to generalize learning to new situations are often quoted as necessary prerequisites for successful psychotherapy, yet deficits in these areas are common in patients with frontal system brain injuries. Deficits in attention, memory, and language will also have an impact on therapy.

Possible changes to the therapy will depend on the patient's needs, deficits, and strengths. Greater repetition or the use of notes or environmental cues may be of some help. Generally, the therapist will take a much more active, and usually proactive, approach by teaching new ways of coping and of managing interpersonal relationships. A highly structured approach is usually best.

Recognition of Patients' Deficits

Recognition of the patient's deficits by mental health workers, family members, and society in general may improve our support of these patients and ultimately lead to improved care. In essence, we need to free ourselves of the belief that disordered personality is somehow these patients' fault—that "they are being manipulative" or that "it's just their personality." Evidence to support the brain's role in defining our personalities may facilitate such understanding. The current status of research on personality disorders may well be analogous to that of schizophrenia research just a few decades ago, when the belief that schizophrenia was the result of maternal overinvolvement led to decreased tolerance of and caring for such patients and their families.

Recognizing the patient's limitations in modulating his or her behavior is not equivalent to endorsing or permitting maladaptive behavior. Establishing firm limits and expecting patients to make efforts toward improvement must continue to be a part of the management of patients with personality disorders. Finally, through psychoeducation, patients and their families may be freed of the constraining effects of guilt, denial of illness, and low self-esteem that currently limit rehabilitation efforts.

Case Report

A full description of this N of 1 study is provided elsewhere (van Reekum and Links 1994). A 21-year-old female university student presented with diagnoses of borderline personality disorder, avoidant personality disorder, recurrent major depressive episodes, and substance abuse. There was a history of family dysfunction, bisibling substance abuse, persistent primary (and later, an onset of secondary) enuresis, and probable learning disabilities. Diagnosed with ADHD as a child, she had received methylphenidate as an adolescent and had reported a positive response to this medication. Attentional difficulties, impulsive behavior, and mood lability were all reported to improve. As an adult, she did not benefit from chlorpromazine, lithium, carbamazepine, valproic acid, lorazepam, or tricyclic antidepressants. She reported modest symptomatic improvement on fluoxetine.

The patient completed a neurodevelopmental history and examination similar to that described earlier in this chapter and agreed to a trial of oral methylphenidate, 20 mg every morning and 10 mg at 4:00 P.M. The active medication was alternated with a placebo (double-blind, provided by the hospital pharmacy at minimal expense) for three randomized treatment pairs. Symptoms and side-effect outcomes were tailored to the patient's presentation.

Results were consistent over each treatment pair; there was approximately a 55% reduction in patient-reported symptoms and a 50% increase in side effects on methylphenidate versus placebo. Physician-rated cognitive skills improved approximately 30% on methylphenidate. Given these data, the patient opted to continue on the medication. This is notable, given issues of noncompliance in patients with borderline personality disorder and other personality disorders, as well as the difficulty in demonstrating a subjective sense of improvement in patients with personality disorders, as opposed to clinician-rated measures of improvement in behavior (Soloff et al. 1986). The subjective changes experienced by this patient included decreased severity and frequency of mood swings, decreased suicidal and self-mutilative thoughts and urges, and decreased anxiety. Side effects included insomnia, suspicious thoughts, sweating, a worsening of enuresis, and racing thoughts.

The long-term efficacy of this medication needs to be closely followed and warrants further study. Although results of an N of 1 study cannot be generalized beyond the individual under study, the results demonstrate the following:

- A careful neurodevelopmental history and examination revealed a treatable, possibly causative, brain disorder.
- The N of 1 study design was useful to ensure valid estimates of efficacy and risk in the individual under study.
- Consideration of the brain's role in determining personality and behavior actually improved this patient's outcome (to date) rather than predicting treatment failure.

Too often, clinicians consider "organic" changes to be nontreatable. Clearly, the causes and sequelae of brain dysfunction are many and varied; involving the brain in one's management considerations presents the possibility of new and novel treatment approaches.

Conclusion

In this chapter, I have presented early evidence suggesting a role for brain dysfunction in the etiology of personality disorders. The need for a full neurodevelopmental assessment follows from this evidence. Assessment techniques reviewed include the neurodevelopmental history; neurodevelopmental syndrome inventories; and the neurological examination, including soft signs, neurological investigations, and neurocognitive testing. Treatment modalities arising from these assessments may include pharmacological management of underlying neurobehavioral disorders, cognitive-behavioral therapies, and modification of existing psychotherapies, along with a greater understanding and acceptance of patients with personality disorders. The need for careful evaluation of treatment outcomes is stressed, and the N of 1 design is recommended.

References

Burke WH, Lewis FD: Management of maladaptive social behaviour of a brain injured adult. Int J Rehabil Res 9:335–342, 1986

Coccaro F, Siever LJ, Klar HM, et al: Serotonergic studies in affective and personality disorder patients: correlates with suicidal and impulsive aggressive behaviour. Arch Gen Psychiatry 46:587–599, 1989

Cowdry RW, Gardner DL: Pharmacotherapy of borderline personality disorder. Arch Gen Psychiatry 45:111–119, 1988

Cummings JL: Clinical Neuropsychiatry. Orlando, FL, Grune & Stratton, 1985

Diller L, Gordon WA: Intervention for cognitive deficits in brain injured adults. J Consult Clin Psychol 49:822–834, 1981

Elliott FA: Historical perspective on neurobehavior. Psychiatr Clin North Am 9:225–239, 1986

Gardner DL, Lucas PB, Cowdry RW: CSF metabolites in borderline personality disorder compared with normal controls. Biol Psychiatry 28:247–254, 1990

Guyatt G, Sackett D, Adachi J, et al: A clinician's guide for conducting randomized trials in individual patients. Can Med Assoc J 139:497–503, 1988

Hollon TH: Behaviour modification in a community hospital rehabilitation unit. Arch Phys Med Rehabil 54:65–72, 1973

Hooberman D, Stern TA: Treatment of attention deficit and borderline personality disorders with psychostimulants: case report. J Clin Psychiatry 45:441–442, 1984

Levin HS: Cognitive rehabilitation: unproved but promising. Arch Neurol 47:223–224, 1990

Linehan MM: Cognitive and behaviour therapy for borderline personality disorder, in American Psychiatric Press Review of Psychiatry, Vol 8. Edited by Tasman A, Hales RE, Frances AJ. Washington, DC, American Psychiatric Press, 1989, pp 84–102

Mesulam MM: Principles of Behavioural Neurology. Philadelphia, PA, FA Davis, 1985

Schwamm LG, van Dyke C, Kiernan RJ, et al: The neurobehavioral cognitive status examination: comparison with the CCSE and MMSE in a neurosurgical population. Ann Intern Med 107:486–491, 1987

Soloff PT, George A, Nathan RS: Progress in pharmacotherapy of borderline disorders. Arch Gen Psychiatry 43:691–697, 1986

van Reekum R: Acquired and developmental brain dysfunction in borderline personality disorder. Can J Psychiatry 38 (suppl):1–7, 1993 van Reekum R, Links PS: *N* of 1 study: methylphenidate in a patient with borderline personality disorder and attention deficit hyperactivity disorder (letter). Can J Psychiatry 39:186–187, 1994

Volpe BT, McDowell FIT: The efficacy of cognitive rehabilitation in patients with TBI. Arch Neurol 47:220–227, 1990

Weintraub S, Mesulam MM: Developmental learning disabilities of the right hemisphere. Arch Neurol 40:463–468, 1983

Wender PH, Reimherr FW, Wood D, et al: A controlled study of methylphenidate in the treatment of attention deficit disorder, residual type in adults. Am J Psychiatry 142:547–552, 1985

Wood RL: Brain Injury Rehabilitation: A Neurobehavioral Approach. Rockville, MD, Aspen, 1987

CHAPTER 5

Comprehending Comorbidity: A Symptom Disorder Plus a Personality Disorder

Paul S. Links, M.D., M.Sc., F.R.C.P.C.

*D*ealing with patients who present with both a symptom disorder and a personality disorder is commonplace in clinical practice. Feinstein (1970) stated that "Although patients with more than one diagnosed disease are frequently encountered in modern clinical practice, the inter-relationships and effects of multiple disease have not received suitable taxonomic attention in clinical science" (p. 455). This statement remains true 25 years later.

This neglect of comorbidity affects our understanding in many areas of clinical medicine (Feinstein 1970). Statistics on the cause of death are usually based on assigning the cause to one particular disorder. Often, however, illnesses interact with one another to cause a patient's demise. Most treatment studies are carried out under "purified circumstances." For example, patients with comorbid diagnoses are often excluded from the study sample. This "purification" process greatly limits the generalizability of findings to many patients seen in clinical practice. The clinical course of a disorder may be affected by the presence of comorbid disorders. For example, the comorbid disorder may shorten the time of detection of a disorder by causing the patient to seek help at an earlier phase of the illness.

In this chapter, I summarize the existing knowledge related to the occurrence of personality disorder with the following symptom disorders: depression, schizophrenia, anxiety disorders, and alcoholism. In reviewing each of the symptom disorders, I discuss the following three issues:

1. Is there an association with specific personality disorders?
2. Is the course of the symptom disorder affected by the comorbid personality disorder?
3. Is the treatment response affected by the comorbid personality disorder?

A case example is presented for each of the symptom disorders. Although it is difficult to generalize from a single case, these examples highlight some general principles to consider when managing a patient's symptom disorder and personality disorder.

The frequency of comorbid symptom disorders with personality disorder diagnoses is largely a direct result of the classification system developed for DSM-III (American Psychiatric Association 1980). The authors of DSM-III purposely created a separate axis for personality disorders to ensure that these disorders were not overlooked, because the clinician's attention is often directed to the usually more florid and acute Axis I symptom disorders. The classification system has encouraged clinicians to make personality disorder diagnoses in patients with symptom disorders.

The concept of comorbidity is fraught with difficulties. The definition of comorbidity varies from one author to another. Feinstein (1970) referred to comorbidity as the presence of an "additional clinical entity that has existed or that may occur during the clinical course of a patient who has the index disease under study" (p. 456). It need not be another disorder; the occurrence of pregnancy, for example, during the course of the index disease might be considered an example of comorbidity. Winokur (1990) believed that comorbidity was the "multiformity of a disease" (p. 570) or the existence of two syndromes or groups of symptoms rather than two distinct diseases. Clarkin and Kendall (1992) defined comorbidity as the occurrence at one point in time of two or more DSM-III-R (American Psychiatric Association 1987) or DSM-IV (American Psychiatric Association 1994) disorders. They called this "cross-sectional comorbidity" (p. 904). Clarkin and Kendall discussed the need to study the sequence and temporal relation of the occurrence of one disorder to another. This they called "longitudinal comorbidity" (p. 904), and they indicated that the cause-and-effect relation between two disorders can be examined in this manner. For purposes of this discussion, the term *comorbidity* is used to refer to the labeling of a symptom disorder and a personality disorder in the same patient at one point in time.

The relation between a comorbid symptom disorder and a personality disorder can be explained in several ways. First, the coexistence of disorders may simply be an artifact of our present classification system. Soloff et al. (1991) noted that DSM-III-R emphasizes the borderline patient's affective symptoms by including criteria such as intense anger, affective instability, recurrent suicidal behavior, and chronic dysphoria. Thus, the overlap with affective disorders results from the inclusion of these affective criteria in the borderline personality disorder diagnosis. Second, the personality disorder may predispose to the development of an Axis I disorder, such as depression. Third, the Axis I disorder may lead to the development of an Axis II disorder. For example, Akiskal (1981) hypothesized that a primary unrelenting or recurrent depressive disorder that begins in childhood or adolescence could lead to a disturbance of personality in adulthood. Fourth, the disorders may be unrelated but occur together. Stein et al. (1993) criticized these models as being "linear" and proposed a "nonlinear" model in which neither the symptom disorder nor the personality disorder is primary but both arise from common causes (biological and/or psychosocial) or develop from independent etiologies but interact in important and complex ways. Much more research is needed to define the concept of comorbidity, and it is likely that the explanation for the coexistence of disorders will vary from one pair of disorders to another.

Major Depression

Clinicians are often faced with patients who meet the criteria for major depression and have a history of a personality disorder. Research confirms this observation; for example, the prevalence of affective disorder diagnoses in patients with borderline personality disorder has ranged from 14% to 83%, depending on the methodology and setting of the research (Akiskal 1981; Gunderson and Phillips 1991). Although much attention had been given to the relation between borderline personality disorder and depression (Gunderson and Phillips 1991; Soloff et al. 1991), Gunderson and Phillips concluded that there is no special relation between the two diagnoses. Other personality disorders have similar rates of occurrence of concurrent or lifetime depression. The association between borderline personality disorder and affective disorder was hypothesized to be due to an underlying shared biological pathogenesis. In general, this hypothesis has not been supported, and the nature of the relation is probably multidetermined, being partly artifact and perhaps shared vulnerabilities in some cases.

The effects of a comorbid personality disorder on the course and treatment response of depression are the following:

- Early age at onset (Charney et al. 1981; Mellman et al. 1992)
- Increased occurrence of suicidal behaviors (Freidman et al. 1983; Pfohl et al. 1984)
- Poor response to treatment (Andreoli et al. 1989; Charney et al. 1981; Pfohl et al. 1984, Soloff et al. 1991)
- Increased risk of recurrence (Akiskal 1981; Shea et al. 1987; Zimmerman et al. 1986)

During acute episodes of depression, patients will endorse more evidence of personality dysfunction, and the successful treatment of the depression will decrease these self-reported levels of personality dysfunction (Joffe and Regan 1989). However, for most patients with a substantiated personality disorder that existed before the acute depressive episode, the successful treatment of depression will, at most, decrease their level of affective distress. These patients are unlikely to be symptom free after treatment. As Soloff et al. (1991) concluded, "pharmacotherapy does not cure character" (p. 25).

Case 1

Ms. A, a 48-year-old woman, had been under almost constant psychiatric care for the last 18 years of her life. She had repeated episodes of severe depression. At these times, she was persistently hopeless, unable to eat or sleep, irritable, agitated, and driven to make potentially lethal suicide attempts. In the hospital, she was demanding, felt entitled to have all of these demands met, and constantly sought the staff's attention.

Ms. A was clear about the cause of her unhappiness that fueled her extreme hopelessness. She had dedicated her life to her elderly parents. Perceiving that she was protecting them from her successful and selfish older brother, she gave up her career and her friendships to fulfill this role. She was content to care for her chronically ill father and to protect her parents from her narcissistic brother. However, at age 30, her rationale for living ended when her mother suddenly died, and shortly thereafter, her father lost his will to live. From that point on, she had demanded that her therapist find her a reason for living.

The patient had received all types of antidepressant medication over the years with only transitory improvement. Meaningful success occurred when several factors came together serendipitously. Her regular therapist of many years suddenly fell ill and was off work for several months. During this period, Ms. A was admitted to a long-stay day program because the local hospital beds were full. She presented to the staff as lost and helpless but needing to maintain herself for her therapist's return. She accepted and, for the first time, persisted with a trial of sertraline, which proved to be of some value. Ms. A noted a significant, although limited, improvement in her dysphoria. When her regular therapist returned, she expressed her awareness of how she had never fully trusted his attempts to help, despite their having worked together for many years. As a result, Ms. A made the conscious decision to no longer embroil the therapy in a hopeless search for hope.

This case illustrates several important principles in the care of patients with symptom disorders and coexisting personality disorders. First, appropriate treatment for the symptom disorder is needed. For example, there is growing evidence that specific serotonin reuptake inhibitors are useful in patients with depression plus borderline personality disorder (Markovitz et al. 1990; Salzman et al. 1992). However, the clinician must solicit the patient's participation in therapy. Often the therapy plays an important but limited role in alleviating symptoms. The patient's expectations of therapy need to be realistic, and both the clinician and the patient need to persist with treatment for several months

before the benefits of the therapy are assessed. Finally, the therapeutic relationship provides a template on which the therapy can
proceed. In this case, the therapist had to accept, internalize, and
rework the patient's projective identification of her hopelessness
and rage. The therapist's sudden illness plus the availability of a
stable alternate caregiver allowed the patient to reinternalize her
rage and hopelessness.

Schizophrenia

Patients with schizophrenia often demonstrate coexisting personality dysfunction. Hogg et al. (1990) ignored the DSM-III exclusion
criteria for making comorbid personality disorder diagnoses in
schizophrenic patients and examined the prevalence of personality disorders in schizophrenia of recent onset. Of the schizophrenic patients they studied, 57% met criteria for an Axis II
diagnosis. Twenty-one percent of the personality disorder diagnoses made by structured interview were for schizotypal personality disorder, and approximately 15% each were for antisocial
and borderline personality disorders.

Jackson et al. (1991) examined the relation of schizophrenia
and other Axis I disorders to Axis II diagnoses. The authors found
that 29% of schizophrenic patients met the criteria for schizotypal
personality disorder, 20% met those for antisocial personality disorder, and 14% met those for histrionic personality disorder. A
higher proportion of schizophrenic patients were diagnosed with
schizotypal and antisocial personality disorder, and a lower proportion were diagnosed with histrionic, dependent, and borderline personality disorders, as compared with those groups with
unipolar affective disorder, mania, and mixed diagnoses.

The nature of this relation has been studied mainly by examining whether the personality disorder is an antecedent to schizophrenia. For example, McGlashan (1983) found that 55% of
patients with schizotypal personality disorder went on to develop schizophrenia during 15 years of follow-up. Researchers
have investigated the possibility of a shared genetic vulnerability
that explains the association between schizotypal and paranoid
personality disorders and schizophrenia (Siever and Davis 1991).
Family studies have consistently found increased rates of schizo-

typal and paranoid personality disorders among the biological relatives of schizophrenic and paranoid psychotic patients, and many biological marker studies have suggested linkages between these disorders (Weston and Siever 1993). The personality dysfunction may also be a consequence of the schizophrenia, and many of these personality traits overlap with the so-called negative symptoms of schizophrenia.

The effects of comorbid personality disorders on the course of schizophrenia are unclear, partly because of the difficulty in defining the existence of a comorbid personality disorder. McGlashan (1983) found a nonsignificant trend for better outcomes in schizophrenic patients with comorbid personality disorders than in patients with noncomorbid schizophrenia.

Comorbid personality disorders may affect compliance with treatment and the establishment of a therapeutic alliance. Therefore, the comorbid personality disorder may have an impact on the course and treatment response of patients with schizophrenia. Frank and Gunderson (1990) carried out a randomized controlled trial of reality-adaptive supportive therapy versus exploratory insight-oriented therapy in nonchronic schizophrenic patients. They found that a good therapeutic alliance predicted remaining in therapy, good medication compliance, and better outcomes at 2-year follow-up.

Although many factors affect the formation of a good alliance, it appears to be more difficult to achieve a good alliance with patients who have personality disorders than with patients who do not have personality disorders (Frank and Gunderson 1990). Terkelsen et al. (1991) suggested attending to personality traits when developing rehabilitation interventions for schizophrenic patients—for example, targeting interventions for the avoidant traits of a schizophrenic patient. Sometimes the behavioral problems that characterize schizophrenic patients with concurrent personality disorders improve when more effective treatment for the schizophrenia is found, including the use of clozapine.

The interpersonal functioning of a patient with schizophrenia can be affected by the negative symptoms that are part of the syndrome, the side effects of neuroleptic medication, the social consequences of the illness, and the psychological reaction to the psychotic process. To establish the diagnosis of a personality disorder, the clinician must specifically inquire about the patient's

interpersonal functioning before or between episodes of schizophrenia. The clinician may need to rely on information from an
informant who had contact with the patient during these times.
The patient's care can be assisted, however, when the clinician
identifies and attends to the coexisting personality disorders in
patients with schizophrenia. The following case illustrates how
difficult it is to separate the two pathological processes.

Case 2

Mr. B, by his 35th birthday, could acknowledge that his life was
greatly improved. He had first presented to a hospital at age 17,
after a SWAT team swarmed his apartment and disarmed him
of several guns and knives. His suspiciousness was extreme, and
he believed that all three of his brothers were out to kill him.

Although the acute episodes of paranoid delusions would resolve, Mr. B continued to be very impulsive. He frequently became embroiled in fights. He was constantly moving from one
apartment to the next. He was often successful in selling himself
to an employer, but a short time later he would perceive some
mistreatment and would quit or be fired. He episodically abused
drugs. Usually he was drawn into drug use by his younger
brother, who was known to be a dealer. He made several impulsive suicide gestures, and he typically was facing a fistful of minor
charges for his behavior.

Despite his antisocial features, Mr. B had always accepted that
he did better on antipsychotic medication and in general was
compliant with treatment. He seemed to trust the clinic staff and
often phoned when he found himself in a crisis. Based on his
trust of the staff, Mr. B accepted a trial of a novel antipsychotic.
He made significant improvement, and his impulsiveness gradually diminished. For the first time, he was able to maintain a relationship with a female copatient. By his 35th birthday, they had
lived together for 2 years, forgoing marriage because of the expense of a wedding.

Although at times people preferred to label Mr. B as antisocial
or as a paranoid schizophrenic, the disorders obviously interact
in important ways. Many of Mr. B's impulsive behaviors appeared to be in response to his underlying paranoid thought content. Aggressive treatment of his symptom disorder led to
important gains. However, this treatment could occur only when

a trusting working relationship could be established with the staff and his psychiatrist.

Anxiety Disorders

Anxiety disorders are discussed separately here to address possible differences in their associations with Axis II disorders. The two major reviews of the relation between anxiety disorders and personality disorders (Mavissakalian 1990; Stein et al. 1993) concluded that there appeared to be no specific connection between panic disorder and agoraphobia and Axis II disorders.

In many cases, patients with panic disorder do not show evidence of comorbid personality disorders. If a patient with panic disorder has an associated personality disorder, most often it will be a dependent or avoidant personality disorder. Social phobia is often found to coexist with avoidant personality disorder (Stein et al. 1993). The overlap between these disorders, however, is partly due to the similarity between the concepts, particularly when the generalized or global subtype of social phobia is considered (Liebowitz et al. 1988). Stein et al. (1993) concluded from their review that many patients with obsessive-compulsive disorder do not have premorbid obsessive-compulsive personality disorders and that other personality disorders are found to coexist with obsessive-compulsive disorder. Again, the nature of the relation between anxiety disorders and Axis II disorders is unclear, but Mavissakalian (1990) contends that panic disorder, agoraphobia, and the coexisting personality traits might best be considered as separate manifestations of a common diathesis.

Two broad generalizations can be made about the effects of comorbid personality disorder on the course and treatment of anxiety disorders. First, patients with comorbid personality disorders tend to be more dysfunctional and to respond less well to treatment for anxiety disorders. Second, the personality functioning often improves with appropriate treatment of the anxiety disorder (Mavissakalian 1990; Stein et al. 1993).

Case 3

Mr. C was age 43 when he came to therapy because of classic episodes of panic. The episodes had increased in frequency but, more important, were interfering at work. Mr. C felt humiliated when he had to rush out of a board meeting in a state of panic. He worked in a highly competitive field and felt extremely vulnerable now that board members had observed his "flakiness."

Mr. C had attempted to get help half a dozen times before. Each time, however, he left therapy because he perceived the therapist as incompetent, simply adopting a "cookbook" approach to his problem. He had always refused medications.

Mr. C came from a successful middle-class family, and he was able to list a series of accomplishments in his business life that he used to compare himself with his same-aged colleagues at work. His personal life was another matter. Mr. C had been married twice, but in both relationships he had been flagrantly unfaithful. Again, Mr. C's major concern was that the mess of his last marriage spilled over to involve colleagues at work. At the time, it came to light that he had been physically abusive to his wife.

Engagement in therapy seemed possible because of Mr. C's concern for his image at work and because he was willing to accept a more "individualized" approach to his problems. Once a strong working relationship was in place, Mr. C accepted more specific treatment for his panic attacks, including medication. In this case, careful attention to the narcissistic personality psychopathology and to the establishment of a working relationship facilitated more specific therapies for the comorbid panic disorder.

Alcoholism

Alcoholism is often diagnosed in patients who also meet the criteria for Axis II disorders. From a community sample, Helzer and Pryzbeck (1988) documented that 15% of alcoholic men, but only 4% of nonalcoholic men, met the criteria for antisocial personality disorder. Thus, alcoholic men were 4 times as likely as nonalcoholic men to receive this diagnosis. Of alcoholic women, 10% met the criteria for antisocial personality disorder, versus only 0.81% of nonalcoholic women. Alcoholic women were 12 times as likely as nonalcoholic women to receive this diagnosis.

Although a strong association has been established between alcoholism and antisocial personality disorder, other personality disorders, such as borderline and avoidant personality disorders, are found to coexist in alcoholic patients. Nace et al. (1983) found that 13% of alcoholic patients admitted to an inpatient substance abuse unit met the criteria for borderline personality disorder. Once again, the nature of the relation between personality disorder and alcoholism is complex and has been the focus of much discussion. Vaillant (1983) argued that the psychological characteristics seen in alcoholic men were the consequences, rather than the cause, of alcoholism.

The existence of comorbid personality disorder does appear to affect the course of alcoholism. Patients with comorbid antisocial or borderline personality disorder appear to have an earlier age at onset of drinking than do noncomorbid alcoholic patients (Nace et al. 1983; Vaillant 1983). When Nace et al. (1986) compared borderline alcoholic patients with nonborderline alcoholic patients, they found that comorbid patients had more extensive histories of drug abuse, suicide attempts, accidents, and legal problems. The borderline alcoholic patients had outcomes comparable to those of nonborderline alcoholic patients at 1-year follow-up, but the comorbid patients showed an earlier return to drug use.

Comorbid antisocial personality disorder appears to be a predictor of poor treatment response of alcoholic patients to alcohol treatment programs (Frances et al. 1984). Our own research suggested that preexisting substance abuse is an important predictor of the continuance of borderline psychopathology during 7–10 years of follow-up (Links et al. 1995). Zanarini (1993) found that among borderline patients with the best outcomes were patients who sustained sobriety over the follow-up period. Prioritizing treatment for alcoholism in a comorbid patient may be critical for reducing the patient's level of personality dysfunction.

Case 4

Ms. D had been attending outpatient appointments for several years. Although she believed she had received little benefit from therapy, she continued to seek help. Ms. D was age 39 years, single, and unemployed. Many years earlier, she had given up her only child for adoption. She was gravely unhappy and furious with her lot in life. Ms. D had been sexually and physically abused as a child. Both her parents had severe alcoholism and had encouraged Ms. D to drink and abuse drugs from age 6 or

7. She remembered that pills and bottles were in every drawer and closet in the house.

Ms. D had been involved in a series of abusive relationships. She had taken numerous overdoses. It seemed that her only sustained commitments were to her mother and aunt, who were frequently emotionally abusive.

Over time, the pattern of Ms. D's behavior became clearer. She typically would miss her standing appointments for several weeks on end. Finally, she would return, feeling very dysphoric, threatening suicide, and requesting admission. Both Ms. D and her therapist began to observe how these episodes were precipitated by a significant increase in her abuse of alcohol and that she would miss her appointments for the several weeks while she was drinking. Finally, when she stopped drinking, her dysphoria intensified and she came to the next scheduled time requesting admission. In retrospect, Ms. D could see that the drinking began when she felt overwhelmed by her rage and fed up with trying to make things better. This rage was often precipitated by negative interactions with her mother.

Ms. D did not see herself as an alcoholic. By her definition, she was nothing like her parents. With gentle persuasion, however, she did come to recognize that the alcohol abuse interfered with therapy and intensified her dysphoria. In addition, her trusted family doctor was an ally in having Ms. D accept the dangers of her drinking. Ms. D refused alcohol rehabilitation because she felt vulnerable and uncomfortable in groups.

At the time of this writing, Ms. D could recognize her pattern of negative emotions, which precipitated her alcohol abuse. Once the abuse had started, she felt too hopeless and ashamed to seek help. Only when her mood deteriorated and she was in crisis did she feel able to return for help. With this knowledge, she had on occasion been able to break the pattern, but she continued to be dependent on alcohol.

This case illustrates the important interactions between the patient's substance abuse and personality pathology. Substance-abusing patients with no borderline psychopathology will often describe positive social situations as high-risk times for abuse. In contrast, a borderline patient will describe a negative emotional state as a risk factor for relapse or increased abuse (Van Horne 1994). As with Ms. D, the effects of alcohol or drug abuse serve only to eventually intensify dysphoria.

Nace (1992) has reported that patients with borderline personality typically fall into one of two categories. Some of these patients readily accept the identity of being "alcoholic" and find great support and benefit from support groups such as Alcoholics Anonymous. Others, however, do not accept this identity and need to examine their alcoholism in the context of a trusting individual therapy relationship. To engage Ms. D in treatment for her alcoholism, the first step was to establish a trusting relationship and then gently to confront the problems resulting from her alcohol abuse. Enlisting the support of significant others, in this case, the patient's family doctor, can be crucial to helping the patient move forward. Over time, this work may lead the patient to develop strategies to prevent relapses of substance abuse.

Conclusion

Some general principles can be followed when working with patients with personality disorders, as outlined here. Symptom disorders often coexist in such patients. As discussed in Chapters 1 and 2, it is important to attend to both the symptom disorder and the personality disorder diagnoses. Specific associations between symptoms and personality disorders can raise the clinician's diagnostic suspicions about the existence of a particular personality disorder. For many of these associations, future research may well determine that comorbidity results from underlying common etiological or pathogenic factors.

In general, patients with comorbid symptom disorders and personality disorders have a poorer prognosis and response to treatment than do patients without comorbid disorders. Treatment usually proves to be of some benefit, however, and in many comorbid patients both disorders are improved after treatment.

Clinicians should actively and aggressively treat coexisting symptom disorders in patients with personality disorders. The clinician must enlist the patient's participation in this venture. The patient's goals for therapy should be matched with the anticipated benefits of therapy. If a patient has more appropriate expectations that treatment will not be totally effective in eliminating symptoms, he or she may be more willing to comply with treatment over longer periods and despite some side effects.

Establishing a working relationship, enlisting the patient's involvement, and awaiting the response to treatment all take time. The clinician must be willing to be patient and to weather some crises while working on these factors. Finally, drawing on the patient's strengths and supports can facilitate each of these steps—the establishment of the working relationship, the patient's participation, and his or her willingness to accept reasonable goals from therapy.

References

Akiskal HS: Subaffective disorders: dysthymic, cyclothymic, and bipolar disorders in the "borderline" realm. Psychiatr Clin North Am 4:25–46, 1981

American Psychiatric Association: Diagnostic and Statistical Manual of Mental Disorders, 3rd Edition. Washington, DC, American Psychiatric Association, 1980

American Psychiatric Association: Diagnostic and Statistical Manual of Mental Disorders, 3rd Edition, Revised. Washington, DC, American Psychiatric Association, 1987

American Psychiatric Association: Diagnostic and Statistical Manual of Mental Disorders, 4th Edition. Washington, DC, American Psychiatric Association, 1994

Andreoli A, Gressot G, Aapro N, et al: Personality disorders as a predictor of outcome. Journal of Personality Disorders 3:307–320, 1989

Charney DS, Nelson JC, Quinlan DM: Personality traits and disorder in depression. Am J Psychiatry 138:1601–1604, 1981

Clarkin JF, Kendall PC: Comorbidity and treatment planning: summary and future directions. J Consult Clin Psychol 60:904–908, 1992

Feinstein A: The pre-therapeutic classification of comorbidity in chronic disease. J Chronic Dis 23:455–468, 1970

Frances RJ, Bucky S, Alexopoulos GS: Outcome study of familial and nonfamilial alcoholism. Am J Psychiatry 141:1469–1471, 1984

Frank AF, Gunderson JG: The role of the therapeutic alliance in the treatment of schizophrenia: relationship to course and outcome. Arch Gen Psychiatry 47:228–236, 1990

Freidman RC, Aronoff MS, Clarkin JF, et al: History of suicidal behavior in depressed borderline inpatients. Am J Psychiatry 140:1023–1026, 1983

Gunderson JG, Phillips KA: A current view of the interface between borderline personality disorder and depression. Am J Psychiatry 148:967–975, 1991

Helzer JE, Pryzbeck TR: The co-occurrence of alcoholism with other psychiatric disorders in the general population and its impact on treatment. J Stud Alcohol 49:219–224, 1988

Hogg B, Jackson HJ, Rudd RP, et al: Diagnosing personality disorders in recent-onset schizophrenia. J Nerv Ment Dis 178:194–199, 1990

Jackson HJ, Whiteside HL, Bates GW, et al: Diagnosing personality disorders in psychiatric inpatients. Acta Psychiatr Scand 83:206–213, 1991

Joffe RT, Regan JP: Personality and depression: a further evaluation. J Psychiatr Res 23:299–301, 1989

Liebowitz MR, Gorman JM, Gyer AJ, et al: Pharmacotherapy of social phobia: an interim report of a placebo-controlled comparison of phenelzine and atenolol. J Clin Psychiatry 49:252–257, 1988

Links PS, Heslegrave RJ, Mitton JE, et al: Borderline personality disorder and substance abuse: consequences of comorbidity. Can J Psychiatry 40:9–14, 1995

Markovitz PJ, Calabrese JR, Schultz SC, et al: Fluoxetine in borderline and schizotypal personality disorder. Paper presented at the annual meeting of the Society of Biological Psychiatry, New York, May 1990

Mavissakalian M: The relationship between panic disorder/agoraphobia and personality disorders. Psychiatr Clin North Am 13:661–684, 1990

McGlashan TH: The borderline syndrome: is it a variant of schizophrenia or affective disorder? Arch Gen Psychiatry 40:1319–1324, 1983

Mellman RTA, Leverich GS, Hauser P, et al: Axis II pathology in panic and affective disorders: relationship to diagnosis, course of illness, and treatment response. Journal of Personality Disorders 6:53–63, 1992

Nace EP: Alcoholism and the borderline patient, in The Handbook of Borderline Patient Disorders. Edited by Silver D, Rosenbluth M. Madison, CT, International Universities Press, 1992, pp 599–610

Nace EP, Saxon JJ, Shore N: A comparison of borderline and nonborderline alcoholic patients. Arch Gen Psychiatry 40:54–56, 1983

Nace EP, Saxon JJ, Shore N: Borderline personality disorder and alcoholism treatment: a one year follow-up study. J Stud Alcohol 47:196–200, 1986

Pfohl B, Stangle D, Zimmerman M: The implications of DSM-III personality disorders for patients with major depression. J Affect Disord 7:309–318, 1984

Salzman C, Wolfson AB, Schatzberg A, et al: Effect of fluoxetine on anger in symptomatic volunteers with Borderline Personality Disorder. Paper presented at the American College of Neuropsychopharmacology, San Juan, PR, December 1992

Shea MT, Glass DR, Pilkonis PA, et al: Frequency and implications of personality disorders in a sample of depressed outpatients. Journal of Personality Disorders 1:27–42, 1987

Siever LJ, Davis KL: A psychobiologic perspective on personality disorders. Am J Psychiatry 148:1647–1658, 1991

Soloff PH, Cornelius J, George A: The depressed borderline: one disorder or two? Psychopharmacol Bull 27:23–30, 1991

Stein DJ, Hollander E, Skodol AW: Anxiety disorders and personality disorders: a review. Journal of Personality Disorders 7:87–104, 1993

Terkelsen KG, Smith L, Gallagher RE, et al: Schizophrenia and Axis II (letter). Hosp Community Psychiatry 42:538, 1991

Vaillant GE: The natural history of alcoholism: causes, patterns and paths to recovery. Cambridge, MA, Harvard University Press, 1983

Van Horne C: Personality disorder and substance abuse. Paper presented at the annual meeting of the American Psychiatric Association, Philadelphia, PA, May 1994

Weston SC, Siever LJ: Biologic correlates of personality disorders. Journal of Personality Disorders 7 (suppl):129–148, 1993

Winokur G: The concept of secondary depression and its relationship to comorbidity. Psychiatr Clin North Am 13:567–583, 1990

Zanarini MC: A two–six year follow-up of borderline outpatients and Axis II controls. Paper presented at the International Congress on the Disorders of Personality, Cambridge, MA, September 1993

Zimmerman M, Coryell W, Pfohl B, et al: ECT response in patients with and without a DSM-III personality disorder. Am J Psychiatry 143:1030–1032, 1986

CHAPTER 6

Rational Pharmacotherapy for Patients With Personality Disorders

Kenneth R. Silk, M.D.

Although the number of studies on the use of psychopharmacological agents in patients with personality disorders is increasing, there is little empirical evidence for the use of a particular pharmacological agent for the treatment of any specific personality disorder (Cocarro 1993; Liebowitz et al. 1986; Stone 1992). There is little consistent, unequivocal information as to which pharmacological agent would be most useful for any specific personality disorder or, furthermore, which pharmacological agent would be most useful for a patient with a given personality disorder in a certain clinical situation or with a specific symptom complex.

For example, it has been reported that a low-dose neuroleptic might be a more effective antidepressant than a tricyclic antidepressant (TCA) for the depression reported by patients with borderline personality disorder (S. C. Goldberg et al. 1986; Soloff et al. 1986a). In a more recent report, Soloff et al. (1993), however, found little evidence that low-dose neuroleptics are more effective than placebo for depression in patients with borderline personality disorder and found that monoamine oxidase inhibitors (MAOIs) may prove to be more effective antidepressants for some patients in this diagnostic category.

Lithium carbonate and carbamazepine, effective antidepressants when used with "pure depressed, noncharacterological" patients, also appear to have some effectiveness in depressed patients with borderline personality disorder, but this effectiveness seems to derive more from the ability of these medications to decrease impulsivity and perhaps lability than from any direct pharmacological effect on mood elevation (Cowdry and Gardner 1988; Gardner and Cowdry 1986; Links et al. 1990). Because of the relation of serotonin to aggression, the selective serotonin reuptake inhibitors (SSRIs) fluoxetine, sertraline, and paroxetine would be expected to have some usefulness in the treatment of patients with borderline and antisocial personality disorders (Cocarro et al. 1989, 1990). Yet good, solid empirical data for the use of SSRIs for the treatment of any personality disorder remains to be presented.

This is not to say that there is no role for the use of pharmacological agents in patients with personality disorders. The scarce empirical research that has been done has been performed primarily in patients with borderline personality disorder, schizotypal personality disorder, or a combination of the two (Soloff 1990). Recent research into social phobia and its relation to avoidant personality disorder may reveal a promising place for MAOIs in these patients (Liebowitz 1993).

In a paper presented in the fall of 1990 at the National Institute of Mental Health's Williamsburg Conference on Personality Disorders, Cocarro (1993) reviewed the pharmacological treatment of patients with personality disorders. He found 11 papers on open trials of medications in patients with personality disorder (Brinkley et al. 1979; Cocarro et al. 1990; Cornelius et al. 1990; Faltus 1984; Hymowitz et al. 1986; Liebowitz and Klein 1981; Markovitz et al. 1991; Norden 1989; Reyntjens 1972; Teicher et al. 1989; Vilken 1964), 4 on controlled trials (Hedberg et al. 1971; Leone 1982; Parsons et al. 1989; Serban and Siegel 1984), and 7 on placebo-controlled trials (Cowdry and Gardner 1988; S. C. Goldberg et al. 1986; Links et al. 1990; Montgomery and Montgomery 1982; Sheard et al. 1976; Soloff et al. 1986a, 1989). These few papers, 22 in all, covered work performed on all of the 11 DSM-III-R (American Psychiatric Press 1987) personality disorders and utilized a variety of pharmacological agents, including neuroleptics, TCAs, MAOIs, lithium, anticonvulsants, anxiolytics, and SSRIs (Cocarro 1993).

Nonetheless, we are gaining greater understanding of some

of the biological mechanisms that may be operating in patients with personality disorders. What is quite intriguing about this biological research is that these studies examine the biological underpinnings of specific dimensions of psychopathology—dimensions that seem relevant across many different personality disorder diagnoses rather than limited to a specific diagnostic entity. Earlier biological research attempted to focus on a specific personality disorder and its similarity to or difference from a specific Axis I disorder (Gold and Silk 1993). Examples of this earlier research are the studies of the dexamethasone suppression test or the onset of rapid eye movement (REM) sleep in patients with mood disorders and those with borderline personality disorder (Baxter et al. 1984; Korzekwa et al. 1993; Lahmeyer et al. 1988; McNamara et al. 1984; Reynolds et al. 1985; Silk et al. 1985, 1988; Sternbach et al. 1983). The recent biological studies, however, have explored the specific dimensions of psychopathology and suggest a relation between each dimension and specific neurotransmitter systems (Siever and Davis 1991).

Cloninger (1987) has proposed classifying personality variants along three dimensions: 1) behavioral activation, or novelty seeking; 2) behavioral inhibition, or harm avoidance; and 3) behavioral maintenance, or reward dependence. Cloninger posited that each of these three dimensions was closely tied to a neurotransmitter system—dopamine to behavioral activation, serotonin to behavioral inhibition, and norepinephrine to behavioral maintenance.

Siever and Davis (1991) expanded on the idea of the relation of dimensions of personality to biological indices. They suggested associations among specific dimensions of personality psychopathology, biological indices, and the three Axis II clusters. They presented four dimensions of personality psychopathology:

1. A *cognitive-perceptual dimension,* which is the primary disturbance found in the odd cluster of personality disorders (schizotypal, schizoid, and paranoid personality disorders) and which may result from disturbances in the dopamine system
2. An *impulsivity-aggression dimension,* which is a dominant disturbance in the dramatic cluster (histrionic, narcissistic, borderline, and antisocial personality disorders) and which may be closely tied to the serotonergic system

3. An *affective instability dimension,* which is also an essential disturbance in the dramatic cluster and which may be closely tied to the cholinergic and noradrenergic systems
4. An *anxiety-inhibition dimension,* which is strongly involved in the anxious cluster (avoidant, dependent, passive-aggressive, and obsessive-compulsive personality disorders) and which may have its underlying disturbance in autonomic function that can be tested through probes such as sodium lactate and yohimbine

Empirical research into the underlying biological processes in patients with personality disorders, as well as specific responses of some borderline patients to pharmacological agents, lends support to the strategy of pursuing dimensions of psychopathology rather than specific diagnoses to better understand the biology of personality disorders. These dimensions may be areas of psychopathology that should be more fully explored and understood in each patient before pharmacological decisions are made (Cocarro 1993). Rather than attempting to elucidate each and every DSM-III-R symptom in order to arrive at an Axis II diagnosis and then making a pharmacological choice based on that specific diagnosis (Klein 1967), there may be greater clinical utility in exploring each of these four dimensions more thoroughly, even though they cut across specific categorical diagnoses. More thorough clinical exploration of each of these dimensions may lead to an informed pharmacological choice based on some putative biological substrate underlying the most prominent pathological dimension (Silk 1994).

These biological studies hold great promise for greater pharmacological specificity (and possibly greater psychopharmacological efficacy) sometime in the future. Amid the current uncertainty, there is important information in the work of Siever and Davis (1991) that may assist the clinician in choosing a pharmacological agent when it appears that a specific dimension of psychopathology is disturbed. Ignoring diagnosis as a specific variable that determines pharmacological treatment (Klein 1967), concentrating instead on disturbed dimensions of psychopathology, perhaps provides the best guidelines to date for treating patients with personality disorders (Silk 1994).

If it appears that, for example, the cognitive-perceptual dimension is the most disturbed, such as when patients show mild to moderate paranoia or odd or idiosyncratic speech or thought (as seen in patients with schizotypal and perhaps paranoid personality disorders) (S. C. Goldberg et al. 1986; Serban and Siegel 1984), then low-dose neuroleptics may be most useful because of the relation of dopamine to cognitive-perceptual disturbances (Siever and Davis 1991). Transient psychotic states or severe or prolonged dissociative episodes (as seen in patients with borderline and perhaps schizotypal personality disorders) may also respond to low-dose neuroleptics (S. C. Goldberg et al. 1986; Soloff et al. 1986a, 1986b).

If the pathological behavior appears to be primarily in the area of impulsivity and aggression, then the serotonergic system (Cocarro et al. 1989; Siever and Davis 1991) may be the neuroendocrine system most disturbed. The SSRIs may be useful in these impulsive and/or aggressive patients (Cocarro et al. 1990; Cornelius et al. 1990; Markovitz et al. 1991; Montgomery and Montgomery 1982; Norden 1989).

Lithium, which can increase postsynaptic serotonergic activity (Linnoila et al. 1983), has been shown to decrease aggression in borderline patients (Links et al. 1990) as well as in some patients with severe personality disorders (Shader et al. 1974). Studies by Siever et al. (1992), in which an increased growth hormone response to intravenous clonidine occurred in patients with personality disorders, suggest a relation between the noradrenergic system and risk-taking, irritability, and impulsivity. Those authors suggest that these traits may culminate in behavior that appears to be a hyperreactive response to environmental stimuli or events. These hyperresponsive patients may be found in most Cluster B disorders (borderline, narcissistic, and histrionic personality disorders), as well as some Cluster C disorders (dependent personality disorder), and this hyperresponsivity may respond to noradrenergic medications such as MAOIs. The MAOIs have been found to be useful in some borderline patients (Cowdry and Gardner 1988; Liebowitz and Klein 1981; Liebowitz et al. 1984; Parsons et al. 1989; Soloff et al. 1993) and have been thought to be particularly useful in hysteroid dysphoric patients, who appear to act out self-destructively in response to emotional triggers (Liebowitz and Klein 1981; Parsons et al. 1989).

Patients who are hyperreactive to the environment may also

respond to minor tranquilizers (Faltus 1984), although there are reports of behavioral dyscontrol when borderline patients are placed on alprazolam (Gardner and Cowdry 1985). Longer-acting benzodiazepines may prove to be less disinhibiting, but caution must be exercised when minor tranquilizers are used in patients who are prone to abuse substances (Dulit et al. 1990).

Further research by Siever and colleagues (Steinberg et al. 1994) has revealed an increased depressive response in borderline and emotionally labile patients when challenged with the cholinesterase inhibitor physostigmine (which essentially increases acetylcholine). This depressive response to physostigmine may help identify depressively labile patients such as are found among those with dependent, borderline, and narcissistic personality disorders. Although Cowdry and Gardner (1988) and Links et al. (1990) have shown that mood stabilizers such as carbamazepine and lithium seem to decrease aggression in borderline patients, it may be that these medications actually decrease impulsivity (i.e., aggression) by stabilizing mood. This stabilization of mood, however, may be different from the antidepressant effect of these medications, because in the studies of Links et al. (1990), Cowdry and Gardner (1988), and Gardner and Cowdry (1986), subjects did not report less depression when taking either of these mood stabilizers.

Anxious cluster patients, especially those with dependent, passive-aggressive, and avoidant personality disorders, may respond to any medication that decreases anxiety through effects on biogenic amines (Yehuda et al. 1994). Thus there may be a place for benzodiazepines, the SSRIs, or the MAOIs among these anxious patients; in particular, the use of MAOIs may have a role in the treatment of patients with avoidant personality disorder (Liebowitz 1993).

Although it appears that some medications are effective in some patients with a given personality disorder or with a particular disturbance in some dimension of psychopathology, it is difficult to predict which patients will respond to which medication or combination of medications. The recommendations outlined here still remain somewhat speculative, and well-done, empirical, controlled studies are needed before these suggestions can become formal guidelines. The responses of patients with personality disorders to medications are often irregular and inconsistent, and they tend to be quite sensitive to side effects. In addition, the role of the placebo response among these patients is unclear. It therefore is clear that prescribing medications to these patients can often become a quagmire of confusing physiological, interpersonal, and other psychological reactions, not only for the patients themselves but also for the psychiatrists who prescribe the medications (Lohr and Benjamin 1992).

In this chapter, I do not review which specific medications have been found to be more or less effective in patients or groups of patients with particular personality disorders. A number of important empirical and open-labeled studies currently present data with respect to pharmacological treatment of some patients with personality disorders (Cocarro et al. 1990; Cornelius et al. 1990; Cowdry and Gardner 1988; Faltus 1984; S. C. Goldberg et al. 1986; Links et al. 1990; Markovitz et al. 1991; Norden 1989; Parsons et al. 1989; Rifkin et al. 1972; Soloff et al. 1986a, 1993). In addition, there are a number of review articles in this area (Cocarro 1993; Cole et al. 1984; Liebowitz et al. 1986; Soloff 1990, 1993; Stone 1992; Zanarini et al. 1988). Unfortunately, most of these studies concentrated on borderline patients, but as stated previously in this chapter, there is scant empirical or other evidence for the effective pharmacological treatment of characterological patients other than those with borderline, schizotypal, and perhaps avoidant personality disorders.

In this chapter, I concentrate on developing a set of methods or procedures that can help clinicians to approach rationally the process of pharmacological treatment of characterological patients. Although much of the information would appear to be most applicable to the pharmacological treatment of borderline or other dramatic cluster patients, these principles can easily be applied across the entire spectrum of diagnoses that comprise the Axis II disorders. I address the following seven issues:

1. Relationship between the therapist and the prescriber
2. Meaning of the medication to the therapist and the prescriber
3. Meaning of the medication to the patient
4. Limitation of the effectiveness of the medication
5. Role of the medication in the overall treatment and treatment plan
6. Lethality of the medication

7. Relation of interpersonal crises and affective storms to the timing of medication initiation or dosage change

After considering these seven issues, I conclude the chapter with some general statements relating to the overall treatment of patients with personality disorders. Consideration of these seven issues within the context of overall patient management is a step toward rational psychopharmacological planning and treatment for patients with personality disorders. It also represents a step away from polypharmacy and pharmacological confusion and disappointment on the part of both the patient and the patient's therapist(s).

Considerations for Rational Pharmacotherapy

Relationship Between Therapist and Prescriber

Although debate remains about the advantages and disadvantages of a therapist-prescriber split in the process of providing a combination of pharmacotherapy and psychotherapy to patients with personality disorders (Koenigsberg 1993), the details of this debate are not covered here. Rather, as changes in health care delivery move forward, especially as they are evolving in the United States, it appears that with increasing frequency psychological treatment will be delivered by a nonphysician provider, whereas pharmacotherapy will be delegated to a physician-psychiatrist (Bradley 1990). This arrangement has been called the *pharmacotherapy-psychotherapy triangle* by Beitman et al. (1984).

When there is an arrangement whereby the prescriber of medication and the deliverer of "psychological intervention" are not the same person, each of these individuals must respect the other's function (Bradley 1990; Woodward et al. 1993). The emphasis in such an arrangement is on whether each provider respects what the other is doing, not whether each respects the other as a person or even as a clinician. As more specifics of mental health care delivery become dictated by third-party providers, organizations that are actually paying the bill, psychiatrists may feel that they are being forced into an uneasy alliance in providing medical backup for therapists whose work they do not respect or do not know much about (R. S. Goldberg et al. 1991). Similarly, therapists may feel uncomfortable if they are limited to referring patients to psychopharmacologists who they feel have little respect for or tolerance of patients' psychological issues.

"In contemporary treatment situations that include a patient, a therapist, a pharmacotherapist, and a pill, the transference issues can become more complex than the landing patterns of airplanes at an overcrowded airport" (Smith 1989, p. 80). As a first step toward a successful combined psychotherapeutic-psychopharmacological effort, it is necessary that both psychopharmacologist and psychotherapist have respect for and some basic understanding of what it is that the other person is trying to accomplish (Docherty et al. 1977), and the two approaches should be coordinated (Koenigsberg 1993).

This does not mean that the psychopharmacologist must be an expert in psychosocial interventions, but he or she should have an appreciation for and some fundamental understanding of the patient's psychological issues. The psychopharmacologist should also have some ability to monitor the degree to which these issues are prevalent or are played out in his or her contacts with the patient concerning medication issues, as well as how those contacts take place.

The psychopharmacologist should make clear and discuss with the psychotherapist his or her beliefs about the efficacy, or the lack thereof, of psychotherapy for the particular personality disorder, as well as for the particular patient under consideration. Psychotherapy for a patient in any diagnostic category cannot proceed constructively if the individual concurrently prescribing psychotropic medications to the same patient does not believe that psychotherapy is a useful undertaking. Other issues should be clarified as well (Woodward et al. 1993), including the following:

- Will between-session phone calls from the patient be permitted during the pharmacological treatment if they are not permitted as part of the psychotherapy treatment?
- How will the pills be prescribed, and in what quantities?
- When the patient requests a change or an increase in dose, will the psychopharmacologist contact the psychotherapist to discuss what might be going on in the psychotherapy at that particular time?

- Will changes in dosage or number of pills prescribed be decided solely by the psychopharmacologist or only after consultation with the other treatment provider?
- How frequently will discussion between the two therapists occur?
- What issues should be directed back to the psychotherapist, and will the psychopharmacologist notify the psychotherapist that issues have been directed back to the psychotherapy?

The following case example illustrates these points:

Case 1

A 21-year-old female college student with a long history of disordered interpersonal relationships complicated by intermittent paranoia was being treated with 50 mg of thioridazine daily. The patient would periodically feel that the therapy was failing and that her therapist was sadistic and deliberately trying to drive her crazy. The therapist and the prescriber agreed to allow the patient to phone or to see the prescriber for short sessions during these crises.

The prescriber maintained the position that these were issues that needed to be worked out with her psychotherapist, and he emphasized his reluctance to try to "medicate away" these particular feelings, which periodically also plagued many of her interpersonal relationships. The prescriber also emphasized that he was always willing to reconsider his decision but that he wanted her to go back and continue to meet as scheduled with her therapist for at least another month. If after that time things had not improved, he would then seriously consider a medication adjustment.

Episodes such as this occurred about twice a year. In the last year of this 5-year therapy, the patient called the prescriber again in a paranoid crisis. She said she knew the prescriber would simply send her back to her therapist to "work it out," and she knew he was right. However, she wanted to call him one last time, for "old times' sake," she said, and tell him that he was correct in making her go back to her psychotherapist to work through the crisis. She currently is not in therapy, is stably employed, remains on thioridazine, and has had limited but healthy interpersonal relationships for the last 2 years.

In a similar manner, the psychotherapist must respect the psychopharmacologist and the intervention of psychopharmacology (Koenigsberg 1993). Although there is little need to be an expert in psychotropic drugs, the psychotherapist should be aware of the specificity and limitations of the psychopharmacological treatment. Thus, the psychotherapist should have some rudimentary knowledge of both the possible therapeutic effects and the possible side effects of the specific medication, and the psychotherapist should be willing to discuss, albeit on a limited basis, the patient's experience (both positive and negative) of taking the medication.

Patients with personality disorders appear to be quite fixed at the transitional object level of functioning (Kernberg 1975, 1984), and thus Axis II patients may be particularly prone to using medications as transitional objects. Both psychotherapist and psychopharmacologist must be aware that patients may use the medications as transitional objects (Winnicott 1953) and that patients' attachment and resistance to changes in medications may seem out of proportion to the actual therapeutic benefit they derived from the medication (Adelman 1985).

These issues should be clarified beforehand between the therapist and the prescriber; otherwise, expectations may run counter to reality, and the combined treatment, particularly with patients with personality disorders, will probably fail. This lack of coordination or understanding with respect to conflicting inpatient models for borderline patients was clearly described by Gordon and Beresin (1983), and a similar conflict can also occur in an outpatient treatment endeavor. It should be made clear to the patient that information will flow freely between the psychopharmacologist and the psychotherapist, and the patient should at the outset sign a release of information that will permit this free exchange of information.

Together the psychopharmacologist and psychotherapist should agree on the perceived efficacy as well as limitations of each of the interventions. They should be able to appreciate that progress among patients with personality disorders is often slow, punctuated by periods of improvement and regression, and that the long-range prognosis is often guarded. This genuine acknowledgment may help prevent the blaming of the other treatment provider when prolonged lack of progress or regression in overall behavior of the patient makes the entire effort frustrating.

It would be useful, both for clarity and from a medicolegal

standpoint, for the therapists to draw up a formal contract between themselves that clearly delineates their respective roles, as well as the expected frequency and range of or limitations on their communication (Appelbaum 1991; Chiles et al. 1991). Should any of these issues change dramatically, the original agreement should be modified. It may also be helpful to inform the patient of the agreement (Chiles et al. 1991).

It should be kept in mind that much of what is diagnosed as personality disorder reflects a group of patients who have chronic maladaptive interpersonal functioning across a wide range of settings. This persistence in interpersonal dysfunction cannot and should not be ignored, dismissed, or denied. Whenever and wherever it occurs during the entire therapeutic process, it should be discussed, not only between the patient's two therapists, but perhaps among the therapists and the patient as well. Transference is not solely reserved for transference-oriented psychotherapy (Beck and Freeman 1990; Goldhamer 1984; Lohr and Benjamin 1992), and "pharmacotherapy is [also] an interpersonal transaction" (Beitman 1993, p. 538).

Much of the mutual cooperation between psychotherapist and psychopharmacologist can be undercut if the patient has been convinced that he or she has a "chemical imbalance." With increasing frequency, patients state that they have been told this. The idea of a chemical imbalance as the sole cause of the patient's difficulties can be particularly problematic for patients with personality disorders, for whom externalization is a major defense mechanism (Kernberg 1975). There is currently little hard evidence that a specific chemical imbalance is responsible for any specific psychiatric disorder or group of disorders. Ultimately, all feelings, cognitions, and behaviors are biochemically mediated, but a more important issue for patients with personality disorders may be how their feelings and cognitions are motivated rather than how they are mediated.

The best approach is one in which the clinician tries not to convince himself or herself or the patient that it is either psychological motivation or chemical mediation alone that is the root of the difficulties (Beitman 1993). Because people are complex beings in whom psychology and physiology play on each other, the best approach is probably one that considers both of these viewpoints rather than tries to finally decide which of the two is paramount (Chiles et al. 1991; Milden 1984). If both psychopharmacologist and psychotherapist believe in this psychological-biological interplay, then it will be easier for the patient to accept that uncertainty, ambivalence, limitation, and cooperation are part of successful everyday existence.

Meaning of the Medication to the Therapist and the Prescriber

As stated earlier, it is important for both the therapist and the prescriber to be aware of the possible effects and limitations of pharmacological intervention in any patient with a personality disorder. These patients defy easy categorizations, despite the slow development and refinement of the empirical base to the Axis II diagnoses, and most pharmacological interventions should be initiated on a trial basis.

In a study by Waldinger and Frank (1989a) of the decision to prescribe medications during the treatment of borderline patients, 65% of the responding psychotherapists thought that pessimism about the patient's progress in therapy was a reason for their decision to consider prescribing medications. Yet rather than consider the situation from a pessimistic point of view, the psychotherapist can view the referral of the patient to the psychopharmacologist as an opportunity for a consultation (Chiles et al. 1991). A good psychopharmacologist should be able to evaluate both the Axis I and the Axis II diagnostic possibilities in the patient, and often a patient with a mild or atypical form of an Axis I disorder can appear to be more characterological than he or she may actually be (Hyler and Frances 1985). The following case example illustrates this point:

Case 2

A 23-year-old law student with a 6-year history of bulimia was referred to the clinic with a diagnosis of borderline personality disorder. The borderline diagnosis had been made because of a 2-year history of suicidal ideation, including cutting behavior, a near-lethal overdose, sarcasm alternating with silence in clinical situations, and the hoarding of medication for a planned overdose during a previous inpatient stay. The psychiatrist believed that, rather than having a personality disorder, this woman appeared to be extremely demoralized over her failure to escape her depression. She slept too much and felt as though she couldn't concentrate or use her intelligence, which had always been an unequivocal ego strength for her. She was bitter and angry over the recent course of her life. A series of seven electro-convulsive shock treatments was very effective in reversing her depression, and many of her "borderline" symptoms disappeared. She remains improved, on antidepressants, 1 year later.

It may be difficult, however, for the psychotherapist to recognize that such a patient may also have a concurrent Axis I disorder, not because of a failure of diagnostic skill on the part of the therapist but rather because of the therapist's own investment in the psychotherapy. Referral for medication often comes not as part of the overall treatment plan but because the psychotherapy has not progressed in the manner hoped, because repeated crises keep interfering with achieving a somewhat smoother course to the therapy, or because of pressure from the patient or the patient's family (Waldinger and Frank 1989). The referring psychotherapist may then develop a feeling of failure, which may be unconsciously conveyed to the patient. On the other hand, if the psychopharmacologist has little respect for psychotherapy or appreciation of the long and arduous process that therapy with personality disorders entails, then the sense of failure will be reinforced by the psychopharmacologist's attitude. If the psychopharmacologist has little genuine belief in the efficacy of medications, then the psychopharmacologist may think that somehow the psychotherapist is saying, "Okay. Now you give it a try. I challenge you to see if your stuff works."

The option of using medication in the treatment of a patient with a personality disorder should not be an afterthought or something that comes up in the course of a treatment that is not going well or has become bogged down. It makes good therapeutic sense to introduce early in the treatment, perhaps as early as when the treatment plan is discussed with the patient, the idea that medications may be quite useful sometime during the course of the treatment (see following case example). It is important to present the idea that the introduction of medications may be useful specifically because the therapy is working well, not because it is failing.

Case 3

A 28-year-old woman with a history of major depressive episodes and schizotypal personality disorder was involved in a particularly acrimonious divorce. Antidepressants had been helpful for her depressions in the past. During the divorce proceedings, the patient did not have a recurrence of her major depression. However, as the divorce approached finalization, she became paranoid and felt that she was unable to think clearly. She was able to distinguish these feelings from the ones that she had had when depressed.

Her therapist's treatment recommendation was for low-dose neuroleptics. At first, she resisted the recommendation, feeling that she would be slipping back if she needed to be on medication again. The therapist worked with her to view the medication as an adjunct to therapy. The therapist also emphasized how the patient, who very often felt dead and unable to experience her own feelings, had been very articulate in describing and differentiating these feelings from those that she had experienced during her depressive episodes. Two milligrams of perphenazine was very helpful to her during the final stages of the divorce proceedings. Two months later, the medication was stopped without a return of the paranoia.

It is most helpful when there is an ongoing professional understanding between the psychotherapist and the psychopharmacologist and when they share responsibility for a number of patients (Smith 1989). Communication can become freer between them. The psychopharmacologist should ask the psychotherapist why he or she wants the medication at this time. Where is the pressure for medications coming from? How does the psychotherapist think the medication will affect the therapeutic relationship? The psychopharmacologist should be able to tell the psychotherapist if he or she believes that the psychotherapist's wishes for the medication are unrealistic, and what might under the best of circumstances be considered a reasonable response to the medications. Mutual respect for what the other does keeps the communication open and useful (Chiles et al. 1991).

Not all treatments, however, have a therapist-prescriber split. In many instances, therapy and medications are given by the same person. In a study by Waldinger and Frank (1989a) of psychiatrists treating borderline patients, only 15% of the psychiatrists chose to split the therapy and psychopharmacology and thus to refer the patient elsewhere for medications. Nonetheless, a clinician who is considering providing the pharmacological as well as the psychotherapeutic treatment should discuss these issues with a colleague if the decision is made to introduce or initiate medication in a patient with a personality disorder.

Meaning of the Medication to the Patient

Although Waldinger and Frank (1989b) have discussed this issue with respect to borderline patients, patients with personality disorders generally may feel that the decision to introduce medications into their treatment means that the psychotherapy has failed or that the psychotherapist has given up on the patient. In some instances, the patient may experience the introduction of medication as a hopeful sign and an additional modality that might help speed the progress of the treatment (Bradley 1990; Gunderson 1984, 1986; Waldinger and Frank 1989a, 1989b).

Understanding what the medication means to the patient is crucial because whenever medication is introduced into any therapy, it has repercussions on the transference process (Goldhamer 1984; Lohr and Benjamin 1992). For patients with personality disorders, the transference can often take on a reality of its own and affect other aspects of the patient's life. Although this does not occur only for patients with personality disorders, it seems to occur with greater frequency and tenacity in these patients than in "neurotic" patients. It is therefore incumbent on both the psychotherapist and the psychopharmacologist to be aware of this complication when medications are introduced into the treatment.

The best way to minimize, but certainly not to eliminate, this transferential reaction is, as mentioned above, to introduce the idea of medication early on in the treatment process. A series of statements that outline how medications might be useful sometime in the course of therapy and how the issue of medications would be approached during the course of treatment should be made at the outset of treatment (Hyland 1991). This series of statements should include remarks relating to the following:

- The introduction of medications does not automatically mean that the treatment is not going well but perhaps may mean that treatment is progressing and entering a new, albeit more stressful, stage.

- Medications will be tried one at a time, and if a particular one does not work after it has been given for a length of time adequate to evaluate its effectiveness, then it will be stopped and replaced by another medication.
- It usually requires a minimum of 3–4 weeks or, in some instances, 3–4 months to fully evaluate the therapeutic effect of a medication.
- A series of medications may need to be tried in sequence, and it is usually better to determine whether one medication can be found that could be effective rather than to keep adding more and more medications at the same time.
- Medications may be useful to treat "ongoing" symptoms but are often not helpful in extinguishing periodic, especially interpersonal, crises.

Often if statements such as these are made at the beginning of treatment, there is a responding dialogue that includes the following issues:

- What might be the indications for medication treatment?
- Who might prescribe the medication?
- What is the chance of becoming "addicted" to a medication once it is begun?
- What might be the effect on one's life or self-image after starting to take psychiatric medication?

In a noncrisis environment, the patient may provide clear indications of what transferential issues might occur if and when medications are introduced. (Of course, the transference paradigms at the beginning of treatment may be different from those arising at the time of the decision to actually add medications, but in many patients the transferential issues may be outlined quite early in the therapy, even if they are not dealt with or interpreted until very much later.) This will allow the psychotherapist to express more fully his or her attitudes about medications at a point early in therapy, when crises may be minimized, transference-countertransference reactions have not fully developed, a spirit of cooperation (either active or passive) is the prevailing mood of therapy, and a clearer and minimally distorted dialogue can take place. However, for the therapist, even a nonmedical therapist, to present a positive but "let's-wait-and-see" attitude, he or she must have some knowledge of what medications can and cannot accomplish.

Limitation of the Effectiveness of the Medication

The therapist should have gained knowledge about what medications can and cannot accomplish at moments of calm, not during periods of crisis, just as issues regarding medications should be presented to patients early in treatment, at moments of calm, rather than in the midst of a crisis. The therapist who first learns about medications during a therapeutic impasse or in the midst of an overpowering affective storm during the therapy will not have a clear and reasonable appreciation of what medications can and cannot do for a patient.

In general, the closer the patient's symptom complex is to the full symptom complex of an Axis I disorder, the greater is the chance that the medication may be effective for some or all of those symptoms. Concurrent Axis I disorders should therefore always be considered throughout the course of therapy, especially when there is a change in the cognitive or affective posture of the patient. Certainly the overlap, in general, between Axis I and Axis II disorders is substantial (Koenigsberg et al. 1985). (Considerations of Axis I and Axis II comorbid states are discussed in Chapter 5.) When there is a clear, unequivocal Axis I disorder present, the medication(s) chosen should conform, in most instances, to the standard treatment for that Axis I disorder, regardless of the comorbid Axis II condition (Stone 1992). Although Axis I patients with comorbid Axis II disorders respond less well and less reliably to pharmacological and other somatic treatments (Charney et al. 1981; Green and Curtis 1988; Zimmerman et al. 1986), this should not deter a serious attempt to identify and treat the comorbid or underlying Axis I disorder with the pharmacological agents usually recommended for the treatment of that disorder. Certain cautions, especially with respect to the treatment of depression in borderline patients with TCAs (Soloff et al. 1986b) or the treatment of anxiety in borderline patients with alprazolam (Gardner and Cowdry 1985), should be considered.

However, the more closely the "symptoms" to be controlled relate to interpersonal issues, emotional lability in the face of rejection, impulsive rage in the face of real or perceived narcissistic injury, or passivity and dependency in the face of opportunity, the greater is the chance that the medications will prove ineffective in these situations.

There are very few good empirical studies of the use of medications in patients with personality disorders. Thus, these statements should be appreciated in the realm of clinical lore, derived from personal clinical experience, and should by no means bear the full weight of clinical fact. Nonetheless, clinical experience as well as clinical facts should be used to present to patients what they can realistically expect from a psychopharmacological trial. Patients should be made to understand that there are no clear-cut rules or explicit predictors of response in these matters. There is only a smattering of empirical data embellished by much clinical lore and intuition, and a successful foray into pharmacological trials demands the cooperation of the patient. Cooperation means compliance with the medication regimen as prescribed, something with which patients with personality disorders appear to have difficulty (Soloff 1993; Waldinger and Frank 1989a). It also means abstaining from substance abuse, reporting side effects, and agreeing not to use the medications as a way to act out against the therapist. This may seem quite idealistic, and it calls to mind a statement made by a borderline patient: "Of course I can rationally agree to anything at this time. However, when I get to feeling despondent, nothing else matters, not even the agreements I have made." Nonetheless, the discussion of medications during periods of calm, both for the therapist and for the patient, has a better chance of being heard with less distortion than if medications are introduced and discussed for the first time during crises or in the midst of a storm of transferential and countertransferential feelings (Koenigsberg 1993). The following case example illustrates this point:

Case 4

A 20-year-old female college student with strong histrionic traits and a family history of alcoholism suddenly began to have panic attacks. They appeared as classic panic attacks that were accompanied by difficulty breathing, headaches, paresthesia, and the feeling that she was surely going crazy. In fact, she was certain that she had been assigned, over a year ago, to see a therapist who worked out of an office located in the hospital so that he would have the hospital close by to admit her when she finally lost her mind.

Given the family history of alcoholism and her fear that she too might become alcoholic, the use of benzodiazepines appeared quite problematic. A suggestion was made that she begin therapy with fluoxetine. The therapist discussed with the patient the possibility that her anxiety and panic symptoms would initially become worse when the fluoxetine was introduced. It was agreed that the fluoxetine would be prescribed at a dose of 10 mg until the patient felt that she was experiencing anxiety no worse than she had without the medication. She was assured that the medication dose would not be increased until she felt ready to increase it. She was also assured that, if the anxiety became much worse after the fluoxetine treatment had begun, there were other medications that could be used, and those medications were discussed as well.

After 4 days of fluoxetine therapy at a dose of 10 mg, the patient requested an increase in the fluoxetine to 20 mg. Although the worst of her panic attacks had ceased after 8 weeks at 20 mg, residual anxiety remained. The fluoxetine dose was increased to 40 mg, and 5 weeks later the patient felt that her anxiety had returned to baseline. The fluoxetine was decreased to 20 mg without an increase in panic or anxiety symptoms.

Role of the Medication in the Overall Treatment and Treatment Plan

The possibility of using medications sometime during the course of treatment should be discussed early in treatment. In fact, it is best for the discussion to take place when the therapist is reviewing the overall goals and limitations of the treatment.

As the other chapters in this volume attempt to make clear, we must reexamine our goals in the treatment of patients with personality disorders. Too often in the past, it would appear that the goal of treatment of these patients was to "cure" them. We must reevaluate what we mean by a cure. To cure someone with a personality disorder cannot imply a goal of completely remaking the person's personality. It is hoped that we will not consider the unrealistic goal of cure; rather, the goals of treatment should be to try to improve the ways in which these patients cope, to help them to develop some increased awareness of their cognitive rigidity and distortions, to assist them in becoming somewhat less affectively labile or passive, and to try to increase the distance between, while reducing the amplitude of, their interpersonal crises (Koenigsberg 1993).

The latter goals seem most realistic, practical, and cost-effective. In any therapy for patients with personality disorders, a series of realistic and limited goals should be set early on in the therapy. The possibility of using medication, its possible therapeutic effects, and its realistic limitations should be introduced within the context of such a discussion of the overall goals and limitations of therapy.

Lethality of the Medication

Unfortunately, many psychotropic medications can be lethal, particularly the TCAs. Carbamazepine, the MAOIs, and the benzodiazepines can also have significant morbidity and mortality associated with overdose. Trazodone and the SSRIs seem somewhat safer than the other classes of medications listed above, and neuroleptics appear to be somewhat safer than the most lethal of the psychotropics. Interestingly, Soloff (1993) believes that overdose among borderline patients appears to be more feared than actually observed. Only five (4.6%) overdoses occurred among 108 borderline patients studied over a period of 4 years, and no overdoses with significant medical consequences occurred among 225 borderline patients over the course of 8 years.

These figures may seem reassuring, but borderline patients are known to have a reasonably high (approximately 10%) rate of successful suicide (Paris 1993; Stone 1990). Patients at highest risk appear to be young (under age 30) males who abuse substances (Montgomery and Montgomery 1982; Stone 1990), but no therapist can ever rest assured that any borderline patient will not overdose with medications.

Fortunately, among all patients with personality disorders, borderline patients probably have the most potential for suicide. The prescribing of any medication for any patient population requires a relationship between the prescriber and the patient. The risks of the medications should be clearly stated, and the patient should be made aware that the process of pharmacological treatment, like psychotherapeutic treatment, can be successful only in the spirit of cooperation. Feelings can be expressed verbally, but when they are acted on, they can lead to serious physical and emotional sequelae.

The potential for suicide must be continually assessed. If the therapist is fearful that the patient may overdose, this issue should be discussed openly. The therapist should not hesitate to ask the patient to bring all medications to a session so that their use and the total amount that the patient is permitted to retain at any given time can be discussed and agreed on. Although the patient may at first object and resist, citing control and trust issues, the patient ultimately cannot deny the concern expressed in the maneuver. I once treated a patient who, when she felt things were getting out of hand, would regularly bring in all her medications and ask me to control them during periods of crisis. When eventually she was able to feel comfortable in keeping her own medication during a crisis, she was able to view herself and her responsibility to herself in a completely different light.

Relation of Interpersonal Crises and Affective Storms to Timing of Medication Initiation or Dosage Change

The introduction of medication into the treatment of a patient with a personality disorder should be done in a controlled manner with much forethought, but it is not always possible to plan ahead in this way. Even when careful plans are made, the interpersonal crises and affective storms that can occur in these treatments, combined with the interpersonal demands or helplessness and passivity of the patient, put enormous pressure on the therapist to do something, to change something, to make the pain go away.

Although medications may be helpful for specific symptoms and symptom complexes, there is no evidence that they change interpersonal functioning. Crises in these patients occur most often in the context of these interpersonal situations or failures, and at this juncture—when the patient is distraught, in pain, perhaps suicidal, and totally pessimistic—there is a great tendency to initiate or to change medications.

Effective pharmacotherapy involves identifying a pattern of reasonably persistent symptoms and choosing the most appropriate medication to address the specific symptom or symptom complex. It is not possible to treat all the symptoms without resorting to polypharmacy, a dangerous and confusing practice, especially among patients in whom psychological motivation and biological mediation is inexorably intertwined. As stated earlier, most psychotropic medications can be lethal if misused. Crises should be weathered by trying not to make sudden changes; patients should be informed that after the crisis has passed, in a calmer moment, the particular pharmacological treatment can be reevaluated (Koenigsberg 1993).

This is not to imply that nothing should be done pharmacologically during a crisis. Perhaps a few doses of a minor tranquilizer may help quell some of the anxiety that accompanies the crisis, but this pharmacological intervention should be very brief and the total number of pills prescribed restricted. There may be a need to prescribe minor tranquilizers on a regular basis, but this decision should not be made at a time of crisis.

Often in the course of psychological treatment of a patient with a personality disorder, the patient comes to a session with an acute crisis, often an interpersonal one. The patient makes a demand that the therapist help him or her solve the crisis that day. Often the patient insists that a decision be made immediately or something disastrous will occur, though what the disaster is remains unclear. The more the therapist wishes to explore the crisis, the more the patient demands immediate advice and a decision from the therapist. Often the session ends without a decision and with the patient angry and unhappy that nothing had been resolved. Although this sounds like a very painful and unempathic situation, it often happens that in the next therapy session no mention is made of the crisis. The situation has somehow passed, nothing disastrous has occurred, and speculation would suggest that a significant transference paradigm was responsible for much of the affect behind the crisis.

A similar situation can occur with respect to medications. A crisis has occurred, something must be done, and the patient insists that the medications are not working and must be changed immediately. Yet by the next session or two, the urgency to change medications has faded, the crisis seems to have disappeared at least for the moment, and therapy proceeds as before. To change medications or dosages in the midst of such demands, particularly when the change is outside of the original thoughtful plan for the pharmacotherapy, often leads nowhere. In fact, the change can lead to progressively higher doses of potentially lethal medicines (Main 1957) or to the practice of polypharmacy, situations that will eventually cloud rather than clarify the clinical picture (Table 6–1).

Table 6–1.   Steps in the pharmacological treatment of patients with personality disorders

Before seeing the patient

1. A nonmedical psychotherapist or a psychiatrist who does not write medications for his or her psychotherapy patients should establish a working relationship with a psychiatrist or psychopharmacologist. The relationship should include

    a. A frank discussion of the nature of their relationship
    b. The limits of and/or sharing of each person's responsibility
    c. The development of an atmosphere wherein each respects the work done by the other

2. A nonmedical therapist should familiarize himself or herself with the range of psychotropic medications available and their main therapeutic and most common side effects.

In the early stages of treatment

1. At the outset of treatment, when the treatment plan and treatment goals are being established, the therapist should bring up with the patient the possibility of pharmacological agents being used sometime during the treatment.

2. When the possibility of medication being used sometime during the treatment is introduced, the therapist should emphasize that

    a. The introduction of medication does not necessarily mean that treatment is not going well.
    b. When medications are tried, they will be tried one medication at a time.
    c. Medication may be helpful for specific symptoms but rarely helps crises or interpersonal interactions.

(continued)

Table 6–1.   Steps in the pharmacological treatment of patients with personality disorders (continued)

When medications are introduced, the psychotherapist and the psychopharmacologist (whether they are the same person or different people) should keep in mind

1. The identification of symptoms or symptom complexes particularly related to Axis I disorders that are medication responsive
2. The meaning of the medication to the therapist and the psychopharmacologist
3. The meaning of the medication to the patient
4. The role of the medication in the overall treatment of the patient, including its role in transference-countertransference reactions
5. The potential lethality of the medication
6. The possibility that a therapist-prescriber split can provide fertile ground to project and act out other splits that occur in the therapy

Caveats to pharmacotherapy

1. All psychotropic medications have some degree of lethality, and some, such as the tricyclic antidepressants, are very lethal.
2. Medication cannot cure or eliminate interpersonal dysfunction.
3. Medication should not, if at all possible, be introduced or changed during times of crisis.
4. Polypharmacy is usually not a useful endeavor and can lead to therapeutic confusion rather than therapeutic clarity.

Conclusion

When medication is prescribed for a patient with a personality disorder, the process of that prescribing becomes a major issue in the management of the patient's symptoms and the treatment. The word *management* should be emphasized because it appears that patients with personality disorders need management as much as they need other aspects of treatment. Management encompasses the entire clinical approach to and overview of the patient.

It seems that nothing that is done with many patients with

personality disorders is simple. Prescribing medications is a complicated process even when there are strong clinical indications that a particular medication might be quite useful in a given patient. The process of prescribing medication to the patient must be managed. This is true whether the pharmacological treatment must be coordinated with the therapist in order to avoid or at least minimize splitting or disagreements, or the therapist and the prescriber are the same person. The pitfall of polypharmacy, and of minimizing the feeling in the patient that the therapist-turned-prescriber has abandoned the more intimate aspects of the psychotherapy for the safer, more distant, perspective of the biological psychiatrist, must be avoided (Gunderson 1984, 1986; Kubie 1971). The successful process of prescribing a medication to a patient with a personality disorder may have as much to do with the "process" of when and how the medication is introduced into the treatment as with the actual choice of the medication itself.

This statement is not meant to imply that words can counteract the effects of medications; it is merely to place forward for consideration the idea that the words used to present and discuss the medication may have as much influence on the outcome of the process of prescribing medication as the actual biological interaction of the medication and the patient. Patients with personality disorders should be told at the beginning of treatment that the suggestion that they take medications may occur sometime during the course of the treatment and that the decision to prescribe medication does not mean that the "talking" part of the treatment is failing or that the patient is getting worse (Waldinger and Frank 1989a, 1989b). Rather, as one gets to know a patient better, one may be able to appreciate more fully which few out of the many symptoms that the patient presents with can become "target" symptoms for psychopharmacological intervention. In the patient with a personality disorder, these target symptoms can be dissected out and followed over time, apart from the rapidly changing affective states and recurrent interpersonal crises.

Although we have no clear biological answers when it comes to understanding the symptoms of patients with personality disorders, we nonetheless should not assume that everything is developmental and should be approached primarily through psychotherapy, a mode of treatment that has not proved to be greatly successful, at least in borderline patients (Waldinger and

Gunderson 1984). If psychotherapy is to be efficacious in these patients, we must find pharmacological as well as psychological "holding environments" (Modell 1976; Smith 1989) so that psychotherapeutic work can proceed more calmly and constructively. This is not to imply that the treatment of these patients should be solely through biological means. These patients will not allow it; they demand great amounts of our time, and no matter how hard we try to avoid transference issues, they nevertheless appear. Thus we must pay attention to the relationship between us and the patients even if we choose the role of psychopharmacologist. Because we may choose a role or treatment that pays less attention to transference-countertransference issues, it does not mean that these issues disappear (Beck and Freeman 1990; Smith 1989).

Although there is always too much transference (a major but unavoidable danger) in the treatment of characterological patients, there can also be too much medication. It may seem useful to treat a patient for all the disturbed symptoms simultaneously, but there is no indication that polypharmacy in these patients is any more successful than in other patients. Furthermore, there may come a point when one must reevaluate all the preceding pharmacological trials and perhaps conclude that there has been no evidence that any medication has shown any real effectiveness in a particular patient. In other words, there may come a point when both the therapist and the psychopharmacologist (embodied in the same person or in two different people) agree that medications just are not working and that all the pharmacotherapy should be stopped (Frances and Clarkin 1981).

The treatment of patients with personality disorders, pharmacological or otherwise, remains empirical. Apart from a few controlled studies on the pharmacological treatment of patients with borderline and schizotypal personality disorders, there is scant information on the pharmacological treatment of patients with other personality disorders. Attempts to effectively treat patients with personality disorders pharmacologically should involve two separate dimensions.

The first dimension is choosing the pharmacological agent. The choice should be made on the basis of a selection of target symptoms for pharmacological change. Interpersonal crises and affective storms cannot be successfully treated pharmacologically at this particular time. Any pharmacological treatment should be tried over a period long enough to evaluate whether the symptom or behavioral dimension chosen for pharmacological intervention has actually improved. We should be modest in our goals and look for a response in clearly defined but limited areas of symptomatology. If one medication does not lead to improvement in the defined, circumscribed area, then the medication should be stopped, new dimensions or symptom targets determined, and a different medication, by itself, tried again for a length of time sufficient for a response to be seen.

The second dimension involves the actual process of prescribing the medication during the course of the treatment. The idea that medication may be used in the treatment should be introduced at the outset of therapy. Decisions must be made as to whether the pharmacotherapy and the psychotherapy are to be dispensed by the same person or by two different people. In prescribing medication, the clinician should take into consideration the following:

- Understanding the relationship between the therapist and the prescriber
- Understanding the meaning of the medication to the therapist and the prescriber
- Understanding the meaning of the medication to the patient
- Understanding the limitation of the effectiveness of the medication
- Understanding the role of the medication in the overall treatment and treatment plan for the patient
- Understanding the lethality of the medication
- Understanding the relationship of interpersonal crises and affective storms to the timing of medication initiation or dosage change

References

Adelman SA: Pills as transitional objects: a dynamic understanding of the use of medication in psychotherapy. Psychiatry 48:246–253, 1985

American Psychiatric Association: Diagnostic and Statistical Manual of Mental Disorders, 3rd Edition, Revised. Washington, DC, American Psychiatric Association, 1987

Appelbaum PS: General guidelines for psychiatrists who prescribe medications for patients treated by nonmedical psychotherapists. Hosp Community Psychiatry 42:281–282, 1991

Baxter L, Edell W, Gerner R, et al: Dexamethasone suppression test and Axis I diagnoses of inpatients with DSM-III borderline personality disorder. J Clin Psychiatry 45:150–153, 1984

Beck AT, Freeman A: Cognitive Therapy of Personality Disorders. New York, Guilford, 1990

Beitman BD: Pharmacotherapy and the stages of psychotherapeutic change, in American Psychiatric Press Review of Psychiatry, Vol 12. Edited by Oldham JM, Riba MB, Tasman A. Washington, DC, American Psychiatric Press, 1993, pp 521–539

Beitman BD, Chiles J, Carlin A: The pharmacotherapy-psychotherapy triangle: psychiatrist, non-medical psychotherapist, and patient. J Clin Psychiatry 45:458–459, 1984

Bradley SS: Nonphysician psychotherapist-physician psychotherapist: a new model for concurrent treatment. Psychiatr Clin North Am 13:307–322, 1990

Brinkley JR, Beitman BD, Friedel O: Low-dose neuroleptic regimens in the treatment of borderline patients. Arch Gen Psychiatry 36:319–326, 1979

Charney DS, Nelson JC, Quinlan DM: Personality traits and disorder in depression. Am J Psychiatry 138:1601–1604, 1981

Chiles JA, Carlin AS, Benjamin GAH, et al: A physician, a nonmedical psychotherapist, and a patient: the pharmacotherapy-psychotherapy-triangle, in Integrating Pharmacotherapy and Psychotherapy. Edited by Beitman BD, Klerman GL. Washington, DC, American Psychiatric Press, 1991, pp 105–118

Cloninger CR: A systematic method for clinical description and classification of personality variants: a proposal. Arch Gen Psychiatry 44:573–588, 1987

Cocarro EF: Psychopharmacologic studies in patients with personality disorders: review and perspective. Journal of Personality Disorders 7 (suppl):181–192, 1993

Cocarro EF, Siever LJ, Klar H, et al: Serotonergic studies in patients with affective and personality disorders: correlates with suicidal and impulsive aggressive behavior. Arch Gen Psychiatry 46:587–599, 1989

Cocarro EF, Astill JL, Herbert JL, et al: Fluoxetine treatment of impulsive aggression in DSM-III-R personality disorder patients. J Clin Psychopharmacol 10:373–375, 1990

Cole JO, Salomon M, Gunderson J, et al: Drug therapy in borderline patients. Compr Psychiatry 25:249–254, 1984

Cornelius JR, Soloff PH, Perel J, et al: Fluoxetine trial in borderline personality disorder. Psychopharmacol Bull 26:151–154, 1990

Cowdry RW, Gardner DL: Pharmacotherapy of borderline personality disorder: alprazolam, carbamazepine, trifluoperazine, and tranylcypromine. Arch Gen Psychiatry 45:111–119, 1988

Docherty JP, Marder SR, van Kammen DP, et al: Psychotherapy and pharmacotherapy: conceptual issues. Am J Psychiatry 134:529–533, 1977

Dulit RA, Fyer MR, Haas GL, et al: Substance use in borderline personality disorder. Am J Psychiatry 147:1002–1007, 1990

Faltus FJ: The positive effect of alprazolam in the treatment of three patients with borderline personality disorder. Am J Psychiatry 141:802–803, 1984

Frances A, Clarkin JF: No treatment as the prescription of choice. Arch Gen Psychiatry 38:542–545, 1981

Gardner DL, Cowdry RW: Alprazolam induced dyscontrol in borderline personality disorder. Am J Psychiatry 142:98–100, 1985

Gardner DL, Cowdry RW: Development of melancholia during carbamazepine treatment in borderline personality disorder. J Clin Psychopharmacol 6:236–239, 1986

Gold LJ, Silk KR: Exploring the borderline personality disorder—major affective disorder interface, in Borderline Personality Disorder, Etiology and Treatment. Edited by Paris J. Washington, DC, American Psychiatric Press, 1993, pp 39–66

Goldberg RS, Riba M, Tasman A: Psychiatrists' attitudes toward prescribing medication for patients treated by nonmedical psychotherapists. Hosp Community Psychiatry 42:276–280, 1991

Goldberg SC, Schulz SC, Schulz PM, et al: Borderline and schizotypal personality disorders treated with low-dose thiothixene versus placebo. Arch Gen Psychiatry 43:680–686, 1986

Goldhamer PM: Psychotherapy and pharmacotherapy: the challenge of integration. Can J Psychiatry 38:173–177, 1984

Gordon C, Beresin E: Conflicting models for the inpatient management of borderline patients. Am J Psychiatry 140:979–983, 1983

Green MA, Curtis GC: Personality disorders in panic patients: response to termination of antipanic medication. Journal of Personality Disorders 2:303–314, 1988

Gunderson JG: Borderline Personality Disorder. Washington, DC, American Psychiatric Press, 1984

Gunderson JG: Pharmacotherapy for patients with borderline personality disorder. Arch Gen Psychiatry 43:698–700, 1986

Hedberg DC, Hauch JH, Glueck BC: Tranylcypromine-trifluoperazine combination in the treatment of schizophrenia. Am J Psychiatry 127:1141–1146, 1971

Hyland JM: Integrating psychotherapy and pharmacotherapy. Bull Menninger Clin 55:205–215, 1991

Hyler SE, Frances A: Clinical implications of Axis I-Axis II interactions. Compr Psychiatry 26:345–351, 1985

Hymowitz P, Frances AJ, Jacobsberg L, et al: Neuroleptic treatment of schizotypal personality disorder. Compr Psychiatry 27:267–271, 1986

Kernberg O: Borderline Conditions and Pathological Narcissism. New York, Jason Aronson, 1975

Kernberg OF: Severe Personality Disorders. New Haven, CT, Yale University Press, 1984

Klein DF: Importance of psychiatric diagnosis in prediction of clinical drug effects. Arch Gen Psychiatry 16:118–126, 1967

Koenigsberg HW: Combining psychotherapy and pharmacotherapy in the treatment of borderline patients, in American Psychiatric Press Review of Psychiatry, Vol 12. Edited by Oldham JM, Riba MB, Tasman A. Washington, DC, American Psychiatric Press, 1993, pp 541–563

Koenigsberg HW, Kaplan RD, Gilmore MM, et al: The relationship between syndrome and personality disorder in DSM-III: experience with 2,462 patients. Am J Psychiatry 142:207–212, 1985

Korzekwa M, Links P, Steiner M: Biological markers in borderline personality disorder: new perspectives. Can J Psychiatry 36 (suppl 1):1–5, 1993

Kubie LS: The retreat from patients: an unanticipated penalty of the full-time system. Arch Gen Psychiatry 24:98–106, 1971

Lahmeyer HW, Val E, Gaviria M, et al: EEG sleep, lithium transport, dexamethasone suppression and monoamine oxidase activity in borderline personality disorder. Psychiatry Res 25:19–30, 1988

Leone NF: Response of borderline patients to loxapine and chlorpromazine. J Clin Psychiatry 43:148–150, 1982

Liebowitz MR: Phenelzine and cognitive behavior therapy in social phobia. Paper presented at the annual meeting of the Psychiatric Research Society, Park City, UT, February 1993

Liebowitz MR, Klein DF: Interrelationship of hysteroid dysphoria and borderline personality disorder. Psychiatr Clin North Am 4:67–87, 1981

Liebowitz MR, Quitkin FM, Stewart JW, et al: Phenelzine v imipramine in atypical depression: a preliminary report. Arch Gen Psychiatry 41:669–677, 1984

Liebowitz MR, Stone MH, Turkat ID: Treatment of personality disorders, in American Psychiatric Association Annual Review, Vol 5. Edited by Frances AJ, Hales RE. Washington, DC, American Psychiatric Press, 1986, pp 356–393

Links PS, Steiner M, Boiago I, et al: Lithium therapy for borderline patients: preliminary findings. Journal of Personality Disorders 4:173–181, 1990

Linnoila M, Virkkunen M, Scheinin M, et al: Low cerebrospinal fluid 5-hydroxyindoleacetic acid concentration differentiates impulsive from nonimpulsive violent behavior. Life Sci 33:2609–2614, 1983

Lohr NE, Benjamin J: When the parameter introduced is medication. Paper presented at the annual Spring meeting of the Division of Psychoanalysis of the American Psychological Association, Philadelphia, PA, April 1992

Main TF: The ailment. Br J Med Psychol 30:129–145, 1957

Markovitz PJ, Calabrese JR, Schulz SC, et al: Fluoxetine treatment of borderline and schizotypal personality disorder. Am J Psychiatry 148:1064–1067, 1991

McNamara E, Reynolds CS III, Soloff PH, et al: EEG sleep evaluation of depression in borderline patients. Am J Psychiatry 141:182–186, 1984

Milden RS: Affective disorders and narcissistic vulnerability. Am J Psychoanal 44:345–353, 1984

Modell A: "The Holding Environment" and the therapeutic action of psychoanalysis. J Am Psychoanal Assoc 24:285–307, 1976

Montgomery SA, Montgomery D: Pharmacological prevention of suicidal behavior. J Affect Disord 4:291–298, 1982

Norden MJ: Fluoxetine in borderline personality disorder. Prog Neuropsychopharmacol Biol Psychiatry 13:885–893, 1989

Paris J: Management of acute and chronic suicidality in patients with borderline personality disorder, in Borderline Personality Disorder, Etiology and Treatment. Edited by Paris J. Washington, DC, American Psychiatric Press, 1993, pp 373–383

Parsons B, Quitkin FM, McGrath PJ, et al: Phenelzine, imipramine, and placebo in borderline patients meeting criteria for atypical depression. Psychopharmacol Bull 25:524–534, 1989

Reynolds CF, Soloff PH, Kupfer DJ, et al: Depression in borderline patients: a prospective EEG sleep study. Psychiatry Res 14:1–15, 1985

Reyntjens AM: A series of multicenter pilot trials with pimozide in psychiatric practice, I: pimozide in the treatment of personality disorders. Acta Psychiatr Belg 72:653–661, 1972

Rifkin A, Quitkin F, Carillo C, et al: Lithium carbonate in emotionally unstable character disorder. Arch Gen Psychiatry 27:519–523, 1972

Serban G, Siegel S: Responses of borderline and schizotypal patients to small doses of thiothixene and haloperidol. Am J Psychiatry 141:1455–1458, 1984

Shader RI, Jackson AH, Dodes LM: The anti-aggressive effects of lithium in man. Psychopharmacology 40:17–24, 1974

Sheard M, Marini J, Bridges C, et al: The effect of lithium on impulsive aggressive behavior in man. Am J Psychiatry 133:1409–1413, 1976

Siever LJ, Davis KL: A psychobiological perspective on the personality disorders. Am J Psychiatry 148:1647–1658, 1991

Siever LJ, Cocarro EF, Trestman RL, et al: The growth hormone response to clonidine in acute and remitted depressed male patients. Neuropsychopharmacology 6:165–177, 1992

Silk KR: Implications of biological research for clinical work with borderline patients, in Biological and Neurobehavioral Studies of Borderline Personality Disorder. Edited by Silk KR. Washington, DC, American Psychiatric Press, 1994, pp 227–240

Silk KR, Lohr NE, Cornell DG, et al: The dexamethasone suppression test in borderline and nonborderline affective patients, in The Borderline: Current Empirical Research. Edited by McGlashan T. Washington, DC, American Psychiatric Press, 1985, pp 99–116

Silk KR, Lohr NE, Shipley JE, et al: Sleep EEG and DST in borderlines with depression. Paper presented at the annual meeting of the American Psychiatric Association, Montreal, May 1988

Smith JM: Some dimensions of transference in combined treatment, in The Psychotherapist's Guide to Pharmacotherapy. Edited by Ellison JM. Chicago, IL, Year Book Medical, 1989, pp 79–94

Soloff PH: What's new in personality disorders? An update on pharmacologic treatment. Journal of Personality Disorders 4:233–243, 1990

Soloff PH: Pharmacological therapies in borderline personality disorder, in Borderline Personality Disorder, Etiology and Treatment. Edited by Paris J. Washington, DC, American Psychiatric Press, 1993, pp 319–348

Soloff PH, George A, Nathan RS, et al: Progress in the pharmacotherapy of borderline disorders: a double-blind study of amitriptyline, haloperidol, and placebo. Arch Gen Psychiatry 43:691–697, 1986a

Soloff PH, George A, Nathan RS, et al: Paradoxical effects of amitriptyline in borderline patients. Am J Psychiatry 143:1603–1605, 1986b

Soloff PH, George A, Nathan RS, et al: Amitriptyline vs haloperidol in borderlines: final outcomes and predictors of response. J Clin Psychopharmacol 9:238–246, 1989

Soloff PH, Cornelius J, George A, et al: Efficacy of phenelzine and haloperidol in borderline personality disorder. Arch Gen Psychiatry 50:377–385, 1993

Steinberg BJ, Trestman RL, Siever LJ: The cholinergic and noradrenergic neurotransmitter systems and affective instability in borderline personality disorder, in Biological and Neurobehavioral Studies of Borderline Personality Disorder. Edited by Silk KR. Washington, DC, American Psychiatric Press, 1994, pp 41–62

Sternbach HA, Fleming J, Extein I, et al: The dexamethasone suppression and thyrotropin releasing hormone tests in depressed borderline patients. Psychoneuroendocrinology 8:459–462, 1983

Stone MH: The Fate of Borderline Patients: Successful Outcome and Psychiatric Practice. New York, Guilford, 1990

Stone MH: Treatment of severe personality disorders, in American Psychiatric Press Review of Psychiatry, Vol 11. Edited by Tasman A, Riba MB. Washington, DC, American Psychiatric Press, 1992, pp 98–115

Teicher MH, Glod CA, Aaronson ST, et al: Open assessment of the safety and efficacy of thioridazine in the treatment of patients with borderline personality disorder. Psychopharmacol Bull 25:535–549, 1989

Vilken MI: Comparative chemotherapeutic trial in the treatment of chronic borderline patients. Am J Psychiatry 120:1004, 1964

Waldinger RJ, Frank AF: Clinicians' experiences in combining medication and psychotherapy in the treatment of borderline patients. Hosp Community Psychiatry 40:712–718, 1989a

Waldinger RJ, Frank AF: Transference and the vicissitudes of medication use by borderline patients. Psychiatry 52:416–427, 1989b

Waldinger RJ, Gunderson JG: Completed psychotherapies with borderline patients. Am J Psychotherapy 38:190–202, 1984

Winnicott D: Transitional objects and transitional phenomena. Int J Psychoanal 34:89–97, 1953

Woodward B, Duckworth KS, Gutheil TG: The pharmacotherapist-psychotherapist collaboration, in American Psychiatric Press Review of Psychiatry, Vol 12. Edited by Oldham JM, Riba MB, Tasman A. Washington, DC, American Psychiatric Press, 1993, pp 631–649

Yehuda R, Southwick SM, Perry BD, et al: Peripheral catecholamine alterations in borderline personality disorder, in Biological and Neurobehavioral Studies of Borderline Personality Disorder. Edited by Silk KR. Washington, DC, American Psychiatric Press, 1994, pp 63–90

Zanarini MC, Frankenberg FR, Gunderson JG: Pharmacotherapy of borderline outpatients. Compr Psychiatry 29:372–378, 1988

Zimmerman M, Coryell W, Pfohl B, et al: ECT response in depressed patients with and without a DSM-III personality disorder. Am J Psychiatry 143:1030–1032, 1986

Introduction to Chapters 7 and 8

*T*he two chapters that follow, "The Script Is Already Written: System Responses to Patients With Personality Disorders" and "The Therapeutic Relationship," are derived from the application of relationship management to the treatment of patients with personality disorders. Relationship management (Dawson 1988) is a model devised primarily for borderline patients. In the following two chapters, however, this model is applied with equal utility to patients diagnosed with other personality disorders or with nonspecific personality disorders, perhaps with the exception of antisocial or sociopathic individuals. For a more complete understanding of the following ideas, the reader is referred to a recently published work on the theory and treatment principles of relationship management (Dawson and MacMillan 1993).

Relationship management is based on an interpersonal analysis of the problems presented to health care professionals, and to the health care system itself, by patients with personality disorders. A choice of a level of analysis need merely be useful in helping patients. Biological reality (i.e., the study of biological mechanisms) is neither more nor less true than social reality (i.e., the study of social processes), although perhaps more easily measured. Researchers may pursue the biological and psychological underpinnings of personality disorder and, for that matter, the definition and categorization (i.e., clustering of traits) of personality disorders, but those people we identify as having personality disorders are, in practice, defined by the interpersonal or social problems they create. Placed more squarely in the interpersonal realm, it could be said that people with personality disorders are so defined because of the problems or social improprieties that emanate from their interactions with a defining other.

That this is so does not negate the possibility that very specific biological or experiential etiological factors will be found in these patients. Finding such specific etiological factors may, in fact, dissolve our current (and always changing) definitions of personality disorder. To an extent, this is happening today as sexual abuse is more frequently being associated with some borderline personality disorders. A movement has developed to redefine such individuals simply as people responding in a "normal" way, or having a "normal" reaction, to the experience of abuse. There is in this interpretation a somewhat antipsychiatry, antimedical tone, but there is no doubt that the diagnosis of personality disorder has negative connotations beyond those of illness itself. The very fact of a psychiatric diagnosis within the context of medical institutions may lead to exuberant overtreatment at times and to rejection at others. It is quite understandable, therefore, if some therapists and some consumer-survivors speak rather disparagingly of the "medical model."

Both the disease concept and the social contract that lie within the medical model when applied to human problems that are defined primarily by cultural and social values cause, as it were, side effects. This must be kept in mind as a cautionary backdrop as we get on with the practical task of trying to understand and help those who seem to be affected by personality disorders.

Many of the tenets of therapy with patients who have experienced abuse resonate well with relationship management, at least in regard to the nature of therapists' contracts with patients. Therapists who work with sexually abused patients know that their patients have had major assaults on their self-system boundaries and therefore need clear, safe, and explicit boundaries in the therapy relationship. These therapists also know that control is a major issue for these patients. Their patients have been victimized. Things outside of these patients' control have been done to them, and yet these patients feel responsible. These patients have also learned to assert control over situations that are or are perceived to be dangerous with whatever means they have at their disposal. Because they were relatively powerless as victims, the control mechanisms of these patients are often those of the powerless: refusal, oppositional behavior, passivity, theater, going on strike, somatization, dissociation, projection, self-abuse, emotional blackmail, and the reenactment of the victim role. Therapists have therefore learned that they must empower these patients and give them control. This is necessary so that they can undergo the tasks of therapy and healing with a sense of security and of mastery over their relationships with therapists, which they do not have to attain through negative behaviors. Relationship management proposes very similar therapy contracts.

Logically, one would work from the specific to the general, from observations and recommendations regarding therapy relationships to inpatient management and then to the patient–health care system. One of the principles of interpersonal and system analysis, however, is that the macro is congruent with the micro, a reflection of and subject to the same processes. For therapists to conceptualize at the interpersonal level, they usually must shelve their well-ingrained notions of linear cause and effect, objective observation (theirs), a psyche organized in vertical layers, and much of the language that describes and regulates these conventions.

The observations and principles of relationship management, therefore, are sprinkled throughout the next two chapters. A mix of micro and macro is presented as the response of the health care system, the multidisciplinary teams of inpatient units, and specific therapist-patient relationships are addressed, ultimately forming, I hope, a consistent whole.

CHAPTER 7

The Script Is Already Written: System Responses to Patients With Personality Disorders

David Dawson, M.D., F.R.C.P.C.

She had been admitted more than 80 times to area hospitals. She was diabetic and overdosed on insulin. She had collapsed once on a bus going past a hospital and on several occasions inside or right outside the emergency room. Two of the hospitals had ruled her unwelcome and forbade her to return. She was admitted to a third hospital after another insulin overdose. When she appeared to have been recovered from this episode, she was given a small amount of freedom. To the horror of the nurses, she smuggled in a utility knife and proceeded to do to herself what they described as a transverse laparotomy. She was placed back on restricted privileges and one-to-one observation.

Another patient had spent 8 months in the psychiatry ward of a general hospital. During this time, she frequently cut herself, spoke of suicide, and demanded to leave. At other times, she appeared energetic and hopeful. The response of the ward staff to her oscillated between control and containment, and support and encouragement. Throughout this period, she was vigorously investigated and treated for an affective disorder. She was then transferred to the psychiatric hospital. There it was believed that she did indeed have an affective disorder but that her difficult behavior was driven by a borderline personality. It was also believed that lengthy and repeated hospitalizations were damaging for her. On discharge, a note was sent to the emergency department advising them not to readmit her. Within days she was back, in crisis, and the afternoon staff of the emergency department requested readmission, not withstanding the note they had received. The inpatient intake worker turned down the request. The resident in the emergency department was brought to an understanding of the situation and tried to comply. Eventually he went off shift. The next morning the intake worker, the attending psychiatrist, and the day shift of nurses, arriving at their usual time, found this woman ensconced on their unit after being admitted during the night.

What is not described in these two case vignettes is the gamut of feelings and attitudes engendered in the staff. Clearly they must have ranged from hope, concern, care, sympathy, and anxiety to irritation, frustration, defeat, hopelessness, hostility, and hatred. Are these patterns of failed health care due entirely to the nature of the illness?

This is probably not the case. However, they do seem to be the natural and predictable consequences of a meeting between medical institutions and someone driven to repeat, in all his or her relationships, certain stylized interactional patterns. Borderline patients are prototypical of this: although described officially by a number of traits and characteristics that imply a disturbed inner state, in actuality they are identified by the distorted interactional patterns they have with others, including health care professionals. People with other personality disorders may be similarly categorized according to their traits and reported experiences, but in practice they are identified by the distorted and troublesome relationships within which they engage others, notably, of course, health care professionals and other helpers.

A person who has been diagnosed with a personality disorder often originally came (or was brought) to a health care institution with an identified problem or problems. These problems may range from suicidality, impulsivity, aggression, alcoholism, and substance abuse to unemployment, anxiety, depression, inability to cope, and posttraumatic stress disorder. Invariably, however, the specter of personality disorder arises when the usual institutional helping strategies fail or are perceived to have failed many times before.

The common way of viewing these counseling and treatment failures is to assume that the patient has a relatively fixed character trait that simply does not yield to advice, persuasion, evidence of its self-defeating properties, insight (either the patient's or the therapist's), or medication. Seen from this perspective, the patient has a character trait that will be expressed within or outside of the context of the health care institution, and the activities of the health care institution are merely ineffective. However, it is often more useful to consider problematic treatment failures as products of the predictable interactions between the patient and the institution.

From this interactional viewpoint, the patient's behaviors are seen not as fixed traits but as negotiating postures. For example, dependency (meaning those behaviors that we tend to see as evidence of dependency) is then seen not as a fixed inner need leading to stereotypical behavior but as a repertoire of behaviors used in interpersonal negotiations. These negotiations have the same objectives as any process-level interpersonal communication: the maintenance or enhancement of "position" and hence of a sense of self. The parameters of position are the same as those being negotiated (sometimes merely being restated) in all interpersonal relationships: relative control, power, dominance, worth, competence, ascendancy, intimacy, and permanency.

Although such relationship negotiations are ubiquitous, for most of us they can be relegated to secondary status or put on hold when other goals are obviously more important. For example, within a simple request one person might make of another person to find a particular file in a filing cabinet, and the second person's response, will be found elements of interpersonal relationship negotiation, if only of affirmation rather than modification or challenge.

History and context can dictate situational parameters or a tradition-bound, role-dependent social contract, and this may serve both participants well, forestalling the need for further negotiation. For example, the social contract of the medical model, with its set rules for reciprocal responsibilities and privileges, spheres of competence, and defined, limited intimacies, will usually facilitate the fulfillment of the goals of both the acutely ill person and the physician without the need for further negotiation about relative control, worth, dominance, etc. (Note, however, that even this traditional social contract between patient and physician is undergoing some adjustment with increased public access to medical information and the "empowerment" of patients, clients, and consumers.)

Those individuals considered to have personality disorders, however, seem driven by primarily interpersonal (process-level) negotiations, even when it would seem prudent for them to put such negotiations on reserve and pay more attention to overt, practical goals and the means to achieve them. For them, content is servant to process. Put another way, these individuals seem to be always in transferential overdrive. Staying within an interpersonal level of observation, it can be said that those people who are considered to have personality disorders are always negotiating with us, using currency appropriate to the context—issues of control, power, worth, responsibility, and competence. (The term *competence* is used here not in its meaning of demonstrated abilities and success but as a position, a role, an assumption.) These attributes, being basically relative, are negotiated against our (the health care system's) apparent or assumed control, power, worth, responsibility, and competency.

The problem lies in the assumed, role-defined, and vigorously exercised attributes of the physician and health care institution: within the traditional social contract of the medical model, the physician must be adequately controlling, ultimately responsible, and extremely competent. Physicians also, of course, have power and are highly valued. A person (patient) seeking to acquire or enhance one or several of these attributes, within the context at hand and relative to the physician's attributes, must then behave in a way that ultimately diminishes the physician's competence, control, power, worth, and responsibility. The physician, and the institution, in other words, must fail. They must fail, not in order to fulfill the overt, stated needs of the patient but to ensure the triumph of the patient's covert negotiations. Unfortunately, the currency used by a patient in these negotiations can be quite self-destructive and dangerous, especially when the physician and the institution remain tenaciously controlling, powerful, responsible, and competent.

In our encounters with people with personality disorders, all is not as it appears to be. On the level of here-and-now interpersonal negotiations (occurring often in subtext, process, behavioral, prelinguistic, and metacommunication), weakness can be strength, failure can be success, total powerlessness can be power, being out of control can be very controlling, and being irresponsible can be masterful. Patients labeled "inadequate and dependent" often leave a trail of failed health care professionals behind them. In this context, within these negotiations, who has been inadequate? The behaviors of the person with an apparently inadequate and dependent personality may actually be mechanisms of power assertion and of interpersonal control, the only mechanisms available to the (self-perceived) powerless, especially in their relationships with health care institutions. Drama, peak experience, inference, affect-laden stories, symbolically loaded language, the burden of our responsibilities, our need to feel in control, our own fear of failure, of incompetence—all these can cloud our perception.

The parameter that many borderline patients appear to be persistently negotiating is control. They may appear to be asking, "Who is in control of the definition of this situation, of myself, and of reality?"

For alcoholic and addicted patients, the issues are often responsibility and worth: "Who is responsible for the trouble I'm in?" Expressed in dialogue, the last line of the play (the script already written) can be read as, "You see, doc, even with your many years of training and your higher education, you couldn't stop me from drinking."

For those people who have been labeled inadequate and dependent, the issues are often competence and power. Despite vigorous application of all the tools at his or her command (advice, encouragement, insight, information, empathy, desensitization, cognitive restructuring, pills), the health care professional fails to get the patient off the couch and into a job or a better relationship. The therapist is rendered a powerless failure, and thus, relatively, the patient acquires power through competently expressed traits of weakness.

Of course, it is difficult to make clear distinctions among control, responsibility, power, worth, and competence; their means of expression and their implications overlap. In practice, it is not that important to discern exactly which parameter is being negotiated, as long as the means are found to alter the negotiations so that patients' assertions or expressions of competence, control, power, self-worth, and responsibility become positive and health promoting rather than self-defeating.

These interpersonal negotiations are carried out in dialogue. The dialogue can often be seen as the externalization of the patient's self-system conflict. This seems especially true for those patients we call borderline. They seem to take a conflict from within their self-perceptions (I am good—I am bad) and enact it in a dialogue with a therapist or health care professional. Typically, such a patient will present one side of his or her conflicted self-system (helpless, incompetent), and the health professional, joining in the dialogue, will assume ownership of the other side (competence). That is, in response, the health professional will assume a posture of competence and offer advice, support, and treatment. This might be helpful, were it not for the fact that this very offering of advice, support, and treatment proposes that the health care professional is competent and in control (the corollary of which is, of course, that the patient is not), and these are the very traits that the patient has come to negotiate. Within the role of *patient* (for those with personality disorders), there is but one way to achieve relative competence and control, and that is to ensure that the health care professional fails.

Boiled down to its skeleton, the usual dialogue may look something like this:

> **Patient:** I am not in control, not competent.
> **Physician:** I am competent; here's some advice (pills) to help you become competent.
> **Patient:** I am still (more) incompetent; the advice (pills) you gave me didn't work (made me worse).
> **Physician:** Okay. I have come to agree with you. You are incompetent and not in control. I will hospitalize you. I am still competent and in control.
> **Patient:** 1) You are wrong. I don't need hospitalization. I am competent; 2) I am even more incompetent (out of control) than that. I will need to be certified, put in seclusion, and closely watched; or 3) You are wrong. I don't need hospitalization, but I am still out of control.

In the hospital, the dialogue or interpersonal negotiation will continue, but now with the added possibility of differential dialoguing, that is, presenting competence and control to one staff member and incompetence to another. In fact, the patient's internal conflict may be externalized into a conflict between staff members. Put another way, the distorting dialogue between the patient and two or more professionals will provoke a parallel distorting dialogue (negotiation) between the professionals.

As this dialogue is tenaciously pursued by the patient, the health care professionals find their positions (also tenaciously pursued) of power, competence, and control shifting to failure and helplessness and followed quickly by anger and rejection. It is also at this point that one can see both sides of the patient's self-system conflict being contiguously expressed and, presumably, experienced.

There is a special kind of satisfying control over others that comes from not being in control of oneself. And there is a special kind of self-esteem, competence, and sense of power that must arise from being so chronically incompetent, hopeless, and helpless that one antagonizes and defeats the best and the brightest health care professionals.

If this is the nature of the relationships sought by people with personality disorders, what more accommodating context could be found than our health care institutions?

The health care professional meets the patients with a personality disorder within the context of an established social contract that defines the privileges and responsibilities of each participant in the ensuing negotiation. The health care professional assumes certain responsibilities for the welfare, and even the behavior, of the patient, who in turn is absolved of certain responsibilities and expectations. In addition, the health care professional is expected to be competent and to do his or her utmost to help. By assigned and assumed role then, and probably by nature as well, the health care professional is compelled to enter into interpersonal negotiations with each patient from a stance of competence, control, power, and responsibility. These are, of course, exactly the parameters the patient has come to negotiate. The script is already written. The dialogue is predictable, as often is, sadly, the outcome.

Psychiatric inpatient wards are usually not beneficial places for people with personality disorders. An inpatient ward embodies the social contract of the medical model in its policies, rules, and expectations, both written and unwritten. This is precisely the kind of interpersonal contract that the person with a personality disorder is driven to contravene. Outcomes are often predictably bad for both the patient and the staff. In addition, it is very difficult to modify this social contract on an inpatient ward, where the complex interdisciplinary organization lies within a larger structure with its overriding set of policies and administrative expectations.

Quite simply, inpatient staff will often apply to the disturbed behaviors and emotional displays of borderline patients (and of people with posttraumatic stress disorder) the same control mechanisms they would use for patients with symptoms of schizophrenia and mania. With the best of intentions in their use of seclusion, medication, and restraints, staff often mimic the cycle of abuse that may have caused the original problems.

I believe that the worst and most dangerous behaviors of borderline patients come about because of, not in spite of, this interactional pattern between patient and health care institution; that subtext negotiations about responsibility and control may drive the delinquent individual to engage in even more delinquent behavior; and that typical negotiations about power and competence with an "inadequate and dependent" patient may ensure even more flagrant displays of helplessness.

An emergency ward, and any inpatient unit, psychiatric or surgical, provides an ideal venue for the narcissistic patient. For these patients, the staff will at first comply with demands ("Am I lovable, am I worthy, and are you loving?" "Yes"); then, as the demands nettle, the staff begin to withhold ("Are you loving?" "Yes, but . . ."). This leads to a progression in the repertoire of the patient and the predictable last act, in which the patient makes outrageous demands while accusing the staff of being hateful, bad, and uncaring, and the staff are vociferously professing love and care while behaving in a hateful, punitive, and rejecting manner.

We cannot ask patients with personality disorders to stop doing what they are doing (at least, we have yet to find a successful way of asking), but we can stop doing what we are doing. These destructive interactional patterns can be changed by

1. Explicitly changing our social contract with patients with personality disorders

2.   Assuming the stance and attitudes of the relationship management approach
3.   Using specific interviewing techniques to maintain that stance

Each case similar to those described in the preceding vignettes can be analyzed within an interpersonal or dramaturgical model. This entails examining the pattern of the patient's relationship with health care institutions over time as well as in any single encounter, avoiding in so doing assumptions of intent or motivation, the language of disease, and psychological models of linear cause and effect. Instead, we should try to discern the process-level relationship parameters being negotiated in each encounter.

When a case is understood in these terms, the treatment team can alter its approach in such a way as to curtail the distorted and destructive interpersonal negotiation about competence, control, and responsibility. This is done by presenting to these patients new social contracts addressing specifically both the parameters they are negotiating and the currency used; for example,

> Joan, you've been admitted to the hospital 15 times now for feeling suicidal, cutting yourself, or overdosing. And in the hospital you have sometimes cut yourself. We haven't been much help to you. So we want to talk this over with you. I'd like to propose that from this point on, you will never be forced to come into the hospital, you'll never again be certified, and should you happen to get certified and arrive in the hospital, you'll be immediately made voluntary. In the hospital, you will always have full freedom and privileges. If you cut or burn yourself, you will be fixed up medically, if you allow this, but nothing else will change. Repeat, nothing else will change. (Or, if you cut yourself or in any other way engage in self-destructive acts, you will be immediately discharged.) We don't want to see you hurt or kill yourself, but it always has been in your power, and always will be, so from this point on, whether you engage in such behavior is entirely up to you. We won't try to stop you. Furthermore, we don't know what pills or programs or kind of talk therapy helps, so from now on you will decide these things. We'll give you what information we have, but you can tell us which medications you want or don't want.

(For a discussion of relationship management for inpatient management, see Dawson and MacMillan 1993.)

The purpose of this new social contract is to eliminate or disqualify certain behaviors as legitimate currency in the ensuing negotiations. These include medication use and abuse, displays of helplessness, suicidal thinking, self-mutilation, and aggression. Within this new social contract, these behaviors are no longer effective.

Clear administrative boundaries must also be drawn for these patients. These boundaries should be administrative in the sense that they are certain, uniformly applied, impersonal, not negotiable, and not (morally) judgmental. They should be based on ethical standards and the tolerance of the therapist and the institution, and they must be enforceable. Examples include the following:

> Whether you drink or abuse drugs between our appointments is up to you, but if you show up for an appointment intoxicated, you will be asked to leave. If you don't leave, a security guard will escort you from the building. The appointment time for the following week will still be available for you.
>
> You decide how much of drug X you wish me to prescribe for you, but the upper limit is 300 mg/day.
>
> I never prescribe narcotics or benzodiazepines; they are addictive. You can probably get them from a number of doctors in town if you want to, but I never prescribe them.

Behind this social contract lie the principles of relationship management. These include a primary goal of doing no harm, or no further harm, and a secondary goal of eliminating the distorted interpersonal relationship between patient and health care system that has been fueling the self-destructive behavior. The third goal is to conduct a corrective therapy relationship within the new social contract.

In a multiagency system, some degree of consistency and coordination would be helpful. This can be achieved through multiagency conferences concerning the more difficult patients and finding a way of applying the new social contract uniformly and consistently. A great deal of time and effort is needed to achieve this, and it seems costly, but not so costly when compared with the alternative: multiple unproductive admissions and years of ineffective and often counterproductive resource utilization.

These conferences should have three stages. The first entails data and perception sharing to determine whether the concepts presented here might be usefully applied. The second stage consists of an attempt to lead the other agencies, therapists, and counselors to the necessary reframing of the problem. Some may come to it quickly, easily adopting the new language of interpersonal negotiation and dropping the perceptions and conceptions that have not been helpful. Others may accomplish this only with difficulty. It does, after all, require them to abandon some steadfast perceptions and language and to question the value of what they have been doing as empathic helpers these many years. A few may not be able to reframe the problem in this way. For personal, professional, or institutional reasons, some cannot come to see that "helping is not always helping." Still others cannot drop their masks of empathy, anxious concern, and responsibility without moving directly to hostility.

A tenet of relationship management is to control those elements that can be controlled and not to attempt to control (or influence) those that cannot be controlled. Thus, therapists or agencies that cannot adopt the new social contract are left alone and considered to be part of the disordered system, on the other side of the dialogue, and the new stance and techniques applied to the patient are now also applied to this agency.

The third stage of these conferences is to apply (negotiate) the new social contract with the patient. This is done with everyone present and in a form that already begins to enact the new social contract. Thus, the patient may decide who is to be there and who is not and what services he or she wishes to obtain from each party. The agency representatives are expected to state, honestly and truly, which services they can and cannot provide. The patient is put in charge. The agencies are expected to respond concretely. Nothing should be left to chance, nothing left vague and abstract.

An example of part of this new multiagency contract and the dialogue to establish it looks something like this:

> **Consultant or case manager:** OK. So am I right, Joan, that you want to see Dr. Smith when you have physical problems, but he'll refer you back to Alice, who will be seeing you once a week, for any emotional or relationship issues?

Joan: Right.

Consultant: Now, in the past you've frequently come into the emergency department with suicidal thinking or an overdose, and they have sometimes admitted you and sometimes tried to not admit you and sometimes certified you and sent you to the hospital involuntarily.

Joan: Sometimes I just need to talk it out.

Consultant: I understand. But the truth is we never know whether to offer you hospitalization or whether it ever really helps. So what would you like the crisis worker to do when you go there and talk about feeling suicidal or have just cut your wrists?

Joan: Well, sometimes I just want to talk, and sometimes I need to be in the hospital.

Consultant: So how about from now on the decision to come into the hospital or just to have a talk and go home will always be up to you. Whatever you decide. No matter whether you've been thinking about suicide or cutting your wrists. Can we do that? (to the crisis service representative)

Crisis service: As long as Joan tells us what she wants.

Joan: Well, sometimes I don't know.

Consultant: So how about if we make the rule that you won't be admitted, ever, unless you ask to be admitted and then, of course, only voluntarily?

Joan: All right.

Consultant: OK. So if you decide to come into the hospital, what do you want to have happen there?

This would now be followed by a dialogue among the consultant, Joan, and the inpatient representative in which Joan would be asked to decide for herself, should she first opt to be admitted, exactly what she would like while in the hospital, and roughly how long she might stay. Of course, the background rules presented to her would include no special observation, no restraints, always voluntary status, her choice of leaving whenever she wants, her choice of medications (with limits), her choice of programs, and no changes or immediate discharge should she engage in any self-mutilating or suicidal behavior (Dawson and MacMillan 1993).

In the setting of this new social contract, concerns will arise in the minds of the various professionals (and perhaps the readers of this book) that this apparent giving over of almost complete control and decision making to the patient could lead to all sorts of abuses: "She'll be in the hospital forever." "She'll ask to be admitted every other week." "She'll come into the hospital and just sit around." "She'll be switching drugs every day."

These fears are unfounded. In fact, the feared excessive length of stay, repeated admissions, refusal to attend programs, and misuse of drugs are far more likely within the traditional social contract. When these and other similar events can no longer be used as negotiating currency, they will vanish.

In the ensuing encounters between this patient and her therapist, crisis workers, and inpatient team members, some specific interviewing techniques are required to maintain and promote the new social contract, to prevent regressive mistakes, and to correct those inevitable mistakes. These techniques ensure that the professionals do not assume (either overtly or subtly) positions that will promote distorted negotiations about control, responsibility, and competence. They will also promote a switch in the pattern of dialogue.

The *switch* refers to a shift on the part of the patient from his or her presenting negative position to something positive; from total hopelessness and incompetence to having a ray of hope, a considered action; from using "I'm out of control" as a means of provoking the controlling responses of helpers to being in control, that is, being in control of oneself in a positive, decisive fashion. (The interview or dialogue techniques used to invoke this switch are discussed in Chapter 8.)

At the beginning of this chapter, a vignette from a rather extreme case was presented, involving 80 admissions, several hospitals, multiple agencies, family doctors, insulin overdoses, and the self-inflicted transverse laparotomy. After several hours of team meetings, all of the principles outlined in this chapter and in Chapter 7 on inpatient management in Dawson and MacMillan (1993) were applied. This patient tested the new contract once, using a self-inflicted wound, and the staff stuck with the agreed-on clause in the contract that "nothing will happen, nothing will change, no special observation, no restraints." The patient then discharged herself to the day program, attended regularly the programs of her choice, took college courses, and remained out of the hospital and has not engaged in any self-destructive behavior for 3 years.

References

Dawson DF: Treatment of the borderline patient, relationship management. Can J Psychiatry 33:370–374, 1988

Dawson DF, MacMillan HL: Relationship Management of the Borderline Patient: From Understanding to Treatment. New York, Brunner/Mazel, 1993

CHAPTER 8

The Therapeutic Relationship

David Dawson, M.D., F.R.C.P.C.

*I*n a psychiatric outpatient clinic some years back, we employed a generous-hearted intake worker who would bring information on new referrals to a large team meeting. People with major psychotic and affective disorders were readily accepted. It was all the others we agonized over. Officially, our questions included, "Will they benefit from therapy? Is there a more appropriate resource? Does this person need counseling, therapy, or a job? Might psychiatry, or 'psychiatrization,' of this person's problem do more harm than good?" We were not Thomas Szasz ideologues, but within every overstatement lies a grain of truth. Absolving badly behaved adolescents of any responsibility via the social contract of the medical model does not improve their behavior. Providing sanctuary and pills for someone using the threat of suicide as a negotiating tool does not extinguish such actions. A diagnosis, pills, and therapy do not usually help someone who is avoiding work, relationship decisions, or responsibility.

Unofficially, the potential therapists were weighing in their minds the kinds of stress and grief each applicant might bring them. "I have a full caseload" was always a good defense. But, of course, these therapists would not be there if they did not have their fair share of empathy, social responsibility, and rescue fantasies. So a good number of difficult applicants were, as the jargon goes, "taken in."

See "Introduction to Chapters 7 and 8," p. 143.

The cases the team resisted most heartily were often those the intake worker worked hardest to sell. A pet phrase was, "I think he really wants help this time." In the team ranks, you could hear words like "personality disorder, sociopath, inadequate, borderline" being muttered.

The therapists were using these terms unprofessionally, pejoratively, and certainly unscientifically. But they were not beginners in the psychotherapy/counseling game and were also simply using shorthand to say something much more complicated and difficult to express in neutral language: "There are pitfalls here. We are already into transference and countertransference overdrive. He may be sincere. He may be motivated." (My favorite definition of *unmotivated* as the word is used in most clinics is, "the patient is not doing what the therapist wants him to do.") "But all is not as it appears to be; an intersubjectivity is clouding our perceptions. In a relationship with this person, I, the therapist, will have to utilize all my resources, and perhaps those of my supervisor, to remain constant, defined, objective, and confined; to accept neither more nor less responsibility than I should; to reasonably balance my duty to my patient with my duty to my patient's children or spouse; to maintain my professional boundaries; to sleep well at night. And after all that, we probably won't get anywhere."

Of course, whether you get anywhere depends on where you planned to go.

So within that simple transaction—the intake worker trying to sell a new patient and the therapists resisting—lie hints of all the problems that can befuddle the relationship of a therapist and a patient with a personality disorder.

When the intake worker opened her mouth to speak, as Arthur Conan Doyle might put it, "the game was afoot." Transference and countertransference were already at work, or, to shift to the framework of the previous chapter, the process level of communication was dominant. Distortions were already apparent. The patient's (applicant's) fantasies of the therapist's magical powers were being passed on by the intake worker, as were the patient's expressions of need and desperation, and even all the irksome hurdles they will mount to thwart the satisfaction of the very needs they profess to have. The therapists were already experiencing a sense of burden. Their language gave this away: "I'm already *carrying* two borderlines." The therapists were experiencing a conflict between their need to be good, helpful, and caring and their dislike of failing and of being unappreciated, responsible for that which they cannot control, and "manipulated."

There are many different kinds of therapy and theories, with greater and lesser scientific validation and plausibility. It would seem as well that what is described about these therapies in journals is not always what actually goes on between patient and therapist, or at least what observers, bringing their own interpretive mechanisms, say is going on. To make matters worse, our therapies, viewed with the wisdom of hindsight, seem as faddish as hula hoops and pet rocks. If nothing more, they underscore our intense need to think that we understand what is going on and our dependence on social context to define, and perhaps limit, what we might think.

Even basic supportive psychotherapy has its downside, as expressed in currently popular terms such as *codependency* and *enabling*. When is being helpful not helpful? When will a positive attitude merely provoke the negative? When does the noncritical acceptance embedded in the social contract of the medical model actually foster a continuation of the problem?

The constant through all of this is, of course, a relationship—between patient and therapist, physician and patient, and always with a third party at hand: the institutional, professional, and cultural context. (The context of an encounter between professional helper and a patient with a personality disorder is discussed in Chapter 7.) In patients with personality disorder, the context may tell us more of what is really going on than the words exchanged or the ostensible intentions and motivations of the participants.

A number of prerequisite questions should be answered before a therapist enters into a relationship with a patient with a personality disorder. First, might such a relationship do more harm than good? Will it promote the very dependency from which the patient *appears* to suffer? Will it enable the patient to transfer blame and responsibility, as he or she is already prone to do? Might the very act of accepting this person's application for being a patient reinforce his or her self-perception of inadequacy? Might in fact a relationship with a competent, controlling, worthy, and caring therapist force this patient to behave worse, even outrageously?

Second, would a different context be safer? Might a self-help group, a club, or a social agency be safer than a medical or psychiatric clinic, where the transactional currencies include pills, suicidal and mutilative behaviors, diagnoses, hospital admission, and notes to employers and licensing bureaus? Where the language is that of illness and disability?

It is interesting to note that groups of psychiatric survivor/consumers, now calling themselves recipients, are using and promoting a variety of unorthodox techniques to promote wellness and to survive relapse. Many of these techniques can be found in the psychiatric literature but seem to achieve potency and legitimacy only when owned by the patients themselves. And this seems to speak volumes about the potential disempowerment of any patient, with or without a personality disorder, of the well-meaning but powerful medical-psychiatric context. Of course, the seriously ill and disabled patient may succumb to a lesser definition of self within the psychiatric context, whereas a patient with a personality disorder will probably fight against it.

The next question is even more difficult. There are limited health care resources. In the most rational of worlds, we would be spending them in the application of efficacious treatment where the burden of illness is greatest and on primary and secondary prevention when that has proved effective. This is part of the context within which a therapist and a patient meet. Therapists must therefore decide how much time and how many resources should be expended in managing patients' personality disorders. What are the goals in doing this? How do we decide when it is not paying off? The latter is perhaps the most pertinent question. Forces other than a rational, thoughtful application of health care resources bring patients with personality disorders into our caseloads. We sometimes "carry" them for years, continuously or intermittently, with no appreciable change. We need to ask what the difference would really be if we were not doing this. Of course none of these questions have definitive answers, but they do provide an examined context within which a clinic and therapist and patient might take the next steps: establishing goals and a contract.

In a sense, the goals are simple. They must be the patient's. More than with other patients, however, the therapist must work to ensure that the goals are truly the patient's, that he or she "owns" them and is responsible for them, and that they do not, at any time, become the therapist's goals *for* the patient.

The therapy contract should be inclusive, clear, and explicit, because it will run counter to and override much of the implicit social contract embedded in the traditional therapist-patient and doctor-patient relationship. In this new contract, the therapist disavows any responsibility for and control or power over the patient's present and future behavior. The therapist will be available at specific times to listen, talk, and offer information. Specific boundaries of the relationship are delineated, as are specific consequences for intolerable behavior occurring during therapy, within the therapist-patient relationship, or within the institution. What the patient does elsewhere is not the therapist's concern.

This may seem cold and heartless, but it need not be. It can be negotiated with warmth and empathy. In the setting of goals and contract with a patient with a personality disorder, the main work of therapy has begun: a corrective relationship. The "inadequate/dependent" patient cannot shift responsibility to the therapist. The "borderline" patient cannot assign power and control to the therapist. The "sociopathic" patient cannot shift blame. The "narcissistic" patient will not receive unconditional love. The addicted patient's habit is his or her own.

The therapist's own goals are limited here. The goals are first, to do no harm or no further harm; second, to provide a managed relationship within which there will be fewer dramatic, dangerous, and self-defeating behaviors than those provoked by a traditional therapy relationship; and third, to provide a context within which the patient may gain control and esteem through positive behaviors.

The purpose of setting explicit goals and creating this type of contract is to manage the already flourishing projections, countertransference and transference, and interpersonal distortions. Through all of this, the therapist is called on to do a great deal of internal work: to not fall prey to the patient's insistent projections and displacements; to not fall prey to his or her own personal and professional needs to be good, wise, helpful, kind, in control, responsible, powerful, and magical; and to "avoid, and avoid again," the traditional assumptions of control and responsibility inherent in the physician-patient relationship.

Inevitably, therapists will fall prey to these forces, but invariably, they are offered second chances. If they have well-tuned "third ears," they will immediately hear the result of their mistake and be able to correct it:

> "Why don't you go back to A.A.?" (the mistake)
> "Bunch of religious nuts. It don't work." (The third ear hears, "Your condescending, controlling advice is bad. You've assumed responsibility for my drinking and have failed.")
> "Yeah, you're right. Sure doesn't work for everybody." ("I was wrong"; the correction)

Specific interviewing techniques are used to establish and maintain this new kind of social contract, to maintain this kind of relationship, and to deflect the patient's persistent attempts to distort the relationship and to force the therapist into traditional role responses and thus into the reenactment of a pathological encounter. In using these techniques, the therapist is waiting for a *switch*. (The switch refers to a shift on the part of the patient from the presenting negative position to something positive, from total hopelessness and incompetence to a ray of hope, a considered action.)

- Slowing down the interview
- Using fewer words
- Using increased silence
- Responding with empathic neutrality
- Assuming a position contrary to assigned role
- Using paradoxical statements

Internal work on the part of the therapist is always necessary to deal with images, fantasies, and an unreasonable sense of urgency, foreboding responsibility, or irritation. To allow time for this internal work and for the therapist to ponder questions of process, the interview can be slowed down. This can be accomplished by responding more slowly, by assuming a relaxed posture, and by inserting natural breaks such as fetching coffee. The purpose of this is to ensure that the process of communication is not overwhelming or controlling the therapist.

A very common pattern of interview dialogue is one in which the therapist's first response is a facilitating utterance ("I see") or empathic reflection ("It certainly sounds . . . "), followed by some elaboration or modification. In the second or third phrase of elaboration, the therapist is most likely to betray the imperatives of the interpersonal negotiation, that is, to respond to his or her own need to offer hope, be clever, demonstrate competence, or maintain control. To test the hypothesis that the process level of communication is paramount, these latter phrases can be consciously withheld. This can be an interesting exercise in itself, because the therapist may then learn to what degree he or she feels compelled to demonstrate competence. The therapist, in withholding, will learn how hard it is to not add those second and third sentences that unnecessarily, and often counterproductively, consist of displays of caring, competence, and cleverness.

There can be comfortable silences in an interview, and there can be very uncomfortable silences. The uncomfortable silences usually occur when either participant has ended a statement in a manner (verbal or nonverbal) that demands a response from the other that is not forthcoming. These are the silences that can be consciously increased in number and duration by the therapist. The patient is left with the ownership of his or her last proposition and must then respond to it. The patient's choices are to repeat it, emphasize it, or modify it. It is the modification (or switch) the interviewer is waiting for:

"Everything's hopeless."
(Silence)
"I just can't go on anymore."
(More uncomfortable silence)
"But I don't want to come into the hospital."
(Silence)
"Maybe I could call my sister."

The subtext in this example is a negotiation of responsibility and competence. The interviewer's silence has left the patient to hold a dialogue with herself. In this segment, the patient arrives at ownership of her positive (competent and responsible) proposition instead of having a dialogue with an active, supportive, and directive therapist in such a manner that she finds she must own and defend the negative while the therapist owns and defends the positive.

The same result can be achieved with responses of benign, neutral empathy—that is, empathic reflection that is devoid of inferences of anxiety, urgency, and responsibility. ("It does sound really bad. Yeah, it does sound hopeless.")

> When I'm brought in to see her for the first time, she's sitting up in an infirmary bed with her newly bandaged legs. Before I'm introduced to her, she plaintively asks, "Do you think I'm hopeless, Doctor?"
> My right brain makes a prompt diagnosis. It ignores my left brain's pleas to take a proper history and do a mental status. I pause only briefly, plop myself into a chair, and say, "Probably."

In this vignette, by answering the question, "Do you think I'm hopeless?" with "Probably," the consultant responded in a manner contrary to his role or attributed assignment in the script. He was expected, at the very least, to ask with empathy, if not pity, why the patient might feel this way, whereupon she would most certainly tell him. Or he was expected to reassure her, in which case she was amply prepared to demonstrate how misinformed he must be. She would then own and defend her position of hopelessness, while he would find himself jumping linguistic hoops to cast a small ray of hope on her situation.

The consultant's answer of "Probably" overturned the dialogue imperative. The patient is left with a dilemma: if she is truly and seriously depressed and genuinely, independently of context, resides solely in a position of hopelessness, then she will perceive the interviewer's response as aloof, but she will not be compelled to counter it. On the other hand, if our hypothesis is right, and the control and relative competence negotiation is more important than her transient inner state, she will be compelled to respond. Because within this framework the negotiation and the thrust, counterthrust, and negation of the interviewer's proposition is more compelling than the actual position assumed, she will feel compelled to respond in a contrary manner. After all, she can achieve a sense of power, worth, and competence within her hopeless state only by demonstrating that the interviewer is even less competent and powerful, by countering his definition of the situation, and by reenacting a pathological relationship. Thus, if the process level of communication is paramount, she must protest his acquiescence. What she actually said, with a somewhat surprised and hurt voice, was, "You're not supposed to undermine a patient's confidence."

This is the switch. Not a bold switch, but a switch nonetheless, because she is now admitting to having confidence (read: hope or competence) and is suggesting that it is the interviewer who might be undermining it. A very good start. He should now probably retract a little, with comments such as, "Well, I don't really know" (empathic neutrality), and leave her with the decision to be hopeless or hopeful.

Some other phrases that less dramatically occupy a position contrary to the assigned attributes of power and competence include "It does sound very messy"; "I haven't any idea what one should do in this situation"; and—a very important phrase for therapists to learn to use with patients with personality disorders—"I don't know."

Finally, if the interviewer harbors no negative countertransference, anger, or hatred toward the patient and no wish to reject, he or she might try a true paradoxical injunction. It must be presented with a subtext of respect, seriousness, and empathy and without a sense of challenge or threat. To the patient in the first vignette, the paradoxical injunction might be presented thus: "Well, you've been admitted to the hospital 27 times, and nothing has seemed to help. And considering how much you've suffered, I'd have to conclude that it is hopeless. If I were in your shoes, I'd give up."

An important aspect of the paradox is to stop talking at this point to avoid countering, modifying, or softening what has just been said. It is this imperative that the therapist should try to leave with the patient. If our hypothesis is right, and the process level of communication is paramount, then the content will follow the imperatives of the process of the relationship negotiation. This patient will be compelled to counter the paradoxical injunction.

Within this managed relationship, a patient can still attend group therapy, social skills training, job training, stress management, anger management, self-help groups, programs for victims of abuse, or whatever else he or she decides to pursue. The patient may also reject these options. It is up to the patient.

The young man had been referred for psychiatric assessment/therapy in order to sanction or terminate his eligibility for continuing disability pension payments. He had been unemployed for several years, had had minor scrapes with the law, and had attended numerous social and job-promoting agencies. The psychiatrist saw him as an angry and oppositional young man, and he, the psychiatrist, assumed a position contrary to that assigned to him.

Psychiatrist: Well, if I were you, I'd stay on the dole.
Patient: Wha' d'ya mean?
Psychiatrist: There's high unemployment, and jobs are scarce; there's no shame in staying on welfare.
Patient: I don't like welfare.
Psychiatrist: Aren't any jobs anyhow.
Patient: I could get a job anytime.
Psychiatrist: Naw. Even if you got a job, it'd be minimum wage down at the mill. No future in it. I'd stay on welfare.
Patient: Like hell. I could get 15 bucks an hour.
Psychiatrist: I doubt it. Even so, it'd be a filthy job, shoving hot steel around, no future at all.
Patient: Four or five good jobs I could get.
Psychiatrist: I doubt it. Unemployment's real high. I've got a good comfortable job, but you're not gonna get anything like this. You oughta stay on the dole.
Patient: Bullshit. Welfare's for losers.

And on the dialogue went, with the young man eventually leaving, saying he was going to prove the psychiatrist wrong, and the psychiatrist saying he would see him again same time next week if he wanted. The next week, the young man canceled his appointment; he could not get off work. There is no long-term follow-up to this single encounter. He may have lost or given up his job shortly thereafter, or he may have been lying. But it did demonstrate the extent to which this patient was driven by power/competency/control negotiations and by the need to be oppositional, and it certainly demonstrated the stance a therapist should assume in any longer relationship.

Another, rather pathetic young man came to the clinic requesting help in that universal and vague way in which many patients with personality disorders ask for help. On the knuckles of four fingers and a thumb were crudely tattooed the letters

L-O-S-E-R. The therapist offered the opinion that he did not think he would be able to help and that he was not sure he would not be simply wasting his time even listening to this would-be patient. The patient retorted that he really needed and deserved help.

> **Therapist:** It'd be a waste of time. You're a loser.
> **Patient:** What? I'm not a loser.
> **Therapist:** Sure you are. You've got it tattooed right there on your fingers, L-O-S-E-R.
> **Patient:** You think I'm a loser?
> **Therapist:** Doesn't matter what I think. You think you're a loser. You got it right there for the world to see.
> **Patient:** Yeah, well, I'm not a loser.
> **Therapist:** Sure you are. You got it right there. L-O-S-E-R. Loser.
> **Patient:** I need help, man.
> **Therapist:** Waste of my time. You think you're a loser, you are a loser. Straight down the drain.
> **Patient:** The hell I am, you bastard.
> **Therapist:** It's right there, L-O-S-E-R.
> **Patient:** I can get rid of that.
> **Therapist:** It's real deep in there.
> **Patient:** It's just ink. I can get rid of it.
> **Therapist:** I doubt you can. But if you do, you can come and talk with me. I've got nothing to offer and I doubt I can help, but you can come and talk.

This patient left in anger and confusion. A few days later, the therapist received a call from a plastic surgeon who told him the young man was in his office telling him he had to get the tattoo off his knuckles. He, the surgeon, would do his best, but he couldn't get it all off.

When this patient returned with abraded knuckles, the therapist remained neutral, pessimistic, and anything but congratulatory and insisted he still had nothing to offer except listening. Besides, he said, he still did not believe his patient had much of a future. He had not worked for months. Obviously, he was still a loser inside. This patient promptly went out and got a janitorial position.

Paradoxical injunctions and the assumption of contrary role positions can be powerful tools in altering the immediate behavior of patients with personality disorders. During a longer relationship, they need to be used sparingly, specifically to overcome blocks and stalemates, and incorporated into a more comprehensive stance of neutral empathy. The assumption behind this is that patients with personality disorders usually achieve power, control, and self-worth through negative, oppositional behaviors. When they experience control and mastery through positive behaviors, even if provoked to do so by a neutral or oppositional therapist, they have learned something. It may become internally motivating. There is certainly ample evidence that many people with personality disorders, at odds with the world for years, eventually come across a positive means to fill the same needs—in counseling school children against drugs and crime, in child care work, as alcohol counselors, or as leaders in consumer/survivor movements.

Another practical approach to therapy for patients with personality disorders that is especially useful in agencies and relationships in which a medical diagnostic system is not used takes the following form: A patient is referred and accepted for therapy/counseling. The therapist applies the usual array of formulations and techniques. These techniques may be rooted in a complex psychoanalytic or behavioral theory or simply patient-centered problem solving. The almost universal components of counseling and therapy include empathy, positive regard, acceptance, support, encouragement, and some form of advice, be it direct and obvious or hidden in subtle forms of modeling, interpretation, clarification, mirroring, and contextual expectation. This latter element is important, because even when therapists think they are practicing nonjudgmental, non-advice-giving therapy, expectations can be found within the very context of therapy, the nature of the agency, the funding body, and the culture. In fact, a patient may be operating in opposition to an unspoken expectation.

At some point, with some patients, the therapist will become aware that the patient is not getting better and is perhaps getting worse, that countertransference is intensifying, and that a sense of burden and frustration is increasing. At this time, it can be useful to assume that the ostensible problems being addressed in therapy are not the overriding problem. The overriding problem may be the counterproductive manner in which this person engages others, including would-be helpers. The therapist can then switch to a relationship management approach, change the contract of therapy, and utilize the techniques described here.

The techniques can be used in a trial to answer the following types of questions:

- If I stop assuming responsibility, will my patient assume some?
- If I stop advising, will my patient come up with his or her own decisions and directions?
- If I stop trying to help, will my patient help himself or herself?
- Are the things that my patient is doing and telling me context dependent; are they actually currencies in a here-and-now negotiation?
- Even if my patient's words reflect an external reality, is he or she stuck simply because I would like him or her to be unstuck?

For the patients described in this chapter, the interpersonal imperative is powerful. As with the two young men described, most patients will be compelled to react to the therapist's change, to the new contract. As a first maneuver, the patient will try to provoke more usual reactions from the therapist (demonstrations of control, competence, wisdom, responsibility). When these are not forthcoming, the patient will switch.

Of course, some patients will instead take their troubles elsewhere, in search of a therapist or physician who will engage them in predictable, repetitive, unproductive, and often harmful negotiations. But then at least we have not done harm or made matters worse. And because the predictable pattern of these relationships usually ends with failure and rejection, the patient may return.

A surprisingly large number of patients stick with a therapist who is applying relationship management when it is applied with some warmth and empathy. They may protest: "I don't know why I come, you're not doing anything for me." "You're the doctor. You should know what drug will help." "You don't care what happens to me." But they stick with it, sometimes firing the therapist one week and reapplying the next. They stick with it because 1) they are locked into a new and challenging interpersonal negotiation in which the imperative to provoke opinions, advice, and responsibility from the therapist is strong and 2) when the therapist refrains from assuming responsibility and giving condescending advice and withholds displays of wisdom and magic, the patients, despite themselves, begin to feel a suffusion of self-worth, confidence, and competence. They are being treated like adults.

To maintain this stance against the onslaught of patients' projections and displacements, colleagues' doubts, institutional anxieties, the therapist's own fantasies of litigation and own needs—the very ones that led to this career choice—is very difficult. The relationship management intervention is often counterintuitive. Practice, experience, peer support, supervision, and consultation are required.

CHAPTER 9

Understanding Patients With Histories of Childhood Sexual Abuse

Paul S. Links, M.D., M.Sc., F.R.C.P.C.
Ingrid Boiago, B.A., R.N.
M. Janice E. Mitton, B.A., R.N., M.H.Sc.

Many patients are coming forward asking for therapy because of a history of childhood sexual abuse. Given that approximately 20% of adult women report a history of incest (Russell 1986), this concern may become a major stimulus for requesting psychotherapy. A growing amount of empirical research has documented that sexual abuse and incest are related to psychological problems in adulthood. Several excellent reviews (Briere and Runtz 1991; Browne and Finkelhor 1986) indicate that women who were abused as children show more evidence of depression as adults, have continuing problems with their parents and difficulty in parenting their own children, are at greater risk to be victimized in their adult life, can have impaired sexual functioning, and are at greater risk for adult psychiatric diagnoses. Within psychiatric populations, borderline personality disorder has been a focus of interest (Brown and Anderson 1991; Bryer et al. 1987; Herman et al. 1989; Links et al. 1988; Ludolph et al. 1990; Ogata et al. 1990; Stone et al. 1981; Westen et al. 1990; Zanarini et al. 1989).

In this chapter, we review the evidence supporting a relation between childhood sexual abuse and borderline personality disorder. We caution therapists about the lack of research that addresses the value of targeting the therapy at the history of childhood sexual abuse and make some suggestions for helping patients with personality disorders who have this history.

Supporting Evidence

The relation between childhood sexual abuse and borderline personality disorder has been receiving attention from both researchers and clinicians. As Judith Herman (1992) has written, this can occur only when a political movement has created the environment in which the scientific evidence can be heard. Because the environment is now receptive to considering an etiological link between disorders such as borderline personality disorder and a history of childhood sexual abuse, it is necessary to ensure that the best possible scientific evidence is put forward to understand this link. Our purpose is to review the existing evidence for an etiological link between childhood sexual abuse and borderline personality disorder. To discuss the etiological link between childhood sexual abuse and borderline personality disorder, we employ the scientific criteria for establishing causality. These same criteria, for example, were used to document the link between cigarette smoking and cancer.

To establish an etiological link, a strong association must exist between the putative causal factor and the disorder, and this association must be shown consistently across the research studies. Perry and Herman (1993) have summarized the research on the prevalence of physical and sexual abuse in borderline patients and note that at least 10 studies have found an association between borderline personality disorder and childhood sexual abuse. They indicate that three of these studies (Herman et al. 1989; Ogata et al. 1990; Zanarini et al. 1989), as well as a recently completed fourth study (Paris et al. 1994) were more rigorously undertaken than others. In these studies, the diagnosis and the history of abuse were independently assessed, and the assessors of the abuse were blind to the clinical diagnosis. Also, the most rigorous studies have established the reliability of the assessment of abuse. In all four studies (Herman et al. 1989; Ogata et al. 1990; Paris et al. 1994; Zanarini et al. 1989), very high rates of sexual abuse were found in borderline patients. The rates vary somewhat depending on the definition of sexual abuse used in the research. If the abuse is confined to events perpetrated by the child's caretakers, then 25%–30% of all borderline patients will endorse such a history. If abuse involves acts perpetrated by any adult, then 75% of borderline patients will endorse this history. From these studies, it is concluded that patients with borderline personality disorder are almost nine times more likely than depressed patients and nearly three times more likely than patients with other, nonborderline personality disorders to report a history of childhood sexual abuse.

For an etiological relation to be established, the correct temporal relation must be shown; that is, the causal factor must precede in time the onset of the disorder. We were unable to find a true experiment of the temporal relation in which a cohort of children who were abused and a nonabused comparison group were followed into adulthood and examined for borderline personality disorder. Without a true prospective study, continuing doubts about the validity of the self-reports of abuse have been voiced. Herman and Schatzow (1987) have provided evidence that over 80% of histories of childhood sexual abuse can be validated or corroborated from other sources. Robins et al. (1985) found that psychiatric patients' childhood memories, particularly those of concrete events, were generally verifiable. Recent concerns for falsification of memory in the context of the psychotherapeutic process need to be addressed. Patients, however, often have reported horrific abuse, and, although the details of the events cannot be verified, the experience of trauma seems undeniable.

The association between childhood sexual abuse and borderline personality disorder should also make good epidemiological sense; that is, it should be consistent with the distribution of the disorder in the community. In fact, the etiological model of childhood sexual abuse does explain the observation that borderline personality disorder is found predominantly in females. Because female children are at much higher risk than male children for sexual abuse, we would expect more women to be at risk for developing borderline personality disorder as adults.

The association should also be specific; that is, a strong etiological relation usually involves a specific cause leading to a specific effect. There is evidence that childhood sexual abuse is very highly correlated with other putative risk factors for adult disorders. Links and van Reekum (1993) and Links et al. (1990) were able to demonstrate that sexual abuse was significantly correlated with physical abuse, foster home placement, nonintact parental marriage, and a measure of parental impairment.

To attempt to address the issue of the specificity of the relation between childhood sexual abuse and borderline psychopathology, four groups of researchers carried out multivariate analyses. Ogata et al. (1990) demonstrated that sexual abuse, rather than physical abuse and neglect, differentiated patients with borderline personality disorder from those with depression. Links and van Reekum (1993), after accounting for the effects of nonintact marital history, physical abuse, separations, foster home placement, and parental impairment, found that sexual abuse was significantly related to borderline psychopathology. Paris et al. (1994) demonstrated that childhood sexual abuse discriminated patients with borderline personality disorder from those with nonborderline personality disorders, whereas other parameters, such as physical abuse, measures from the Parental Bonding Index, and separation or loss, did not differentiate the groups. Zanarini et al. (1993) found that sexual abuse by a male caretaker and sexual abuse by a male noncaretaker significantly differentiated borderline patients from patients with other personality disorders. Emotional withdrawal by a male caretaker and a lack of a real emotional relationship with a female caretaker also differentiated the different diagnostic groups. Therefore, this research supports the hypothesis that childhood sexual abuse has a unique relation to borderline psychopathology that is not explained by a confounding relation with other putative causal factors.

The next question is whether the childhood sexual abuse leads to a specific effect in regard to diagnosis. Community samples of women who were sexually abused in childhood report symptoms such as suicide attempts, substance abuse, emotional instability, unstable relationships, and repeated sexual victimization in adulthood. These symptoms are similar to those that contribute to the diagnosis of borderline personality disorder. However, many other disorders, including eating disorders, substance abuse, and dissociative disorders, have been implicated as having a relation to childhood sexual abuse. The strength of the association between childhood sexual abuse and borderline personality disorder is attenuated when compared with closely related disorders.

The specificity of the relation of childhood sexual abuse to borderline psychopathology appears to be explained by certain symptoms. Ogata et al. (1990) found that the symptoms most strongly related to childhood sexual abuse were derealization and chronic dysphoria. Links et al. (1990) found that borderline patients who had been abused showed more self-mutilation, substance abuse, derealization, and depersonalization than did nonabused borderline patients. Herman et al. (1989) demonstrated that dissociative symptoms were related to childhood sexual abuse, even after controlling for the presence of borderline personality disorder. Paris and colleagues (Paris et al. 1994; Zweig-Frank et al. 1994) could not replicate the relation between dissociative symptoms and childhood sexual abuse. In fact, these authors found that the presence of dissociative symptoms seemed to be uniquely related to the borderline personality disorder and were not explained by a history of childhood sexual abuse.

A dose-response relation, or an increased risk of the disease with increased exposure to the putative cause, strengthens the evidence of an etiological relation. Several investigators have examined whether the severity of exposure is related to borderline psychopathology. In their initial study, Zanarini et al. (1989) found that severe and repetitious abuse was related most significantly to borderline personality disorder. Paris et al. (1994), in their careful study of the parameters of abuse, found that penetration and multiple perpetrators (two measures of severe abuse) were related to borderline personality disorder. Herman et al. (1989) found that the number of perpetrators and the duration of abuse were correlated to borderline psychopathology but not to antisocial or schizotypal pathology. Bryer et al. (1987) found that a combination of physical and sexual abuse was the best predictor and was more strongly correlated with borderline psychopathology than was either of the types of abuse alone.

If the association between childhood sexual abuse and borderline personality disorder is analogous to another established etiological model, this will support the proposed etiological relation. Judith Herman (1992) explained borderline personality disorder as a "complex posttraumatic stress disorder" (p. 119). Herman suggested that the trauma of childhood sexual abuse leads to long-lasting effects that in adulthood have many similarities to a complex posttraumatic stress disorder. The withdrawal and overreactivity that are characteristic of patients with posttraumatic stress disorder explain many of the features of borderline personality disorder. Herman has outlined a model of therapy based on her analogy (1992). Rutter and Giller (1984) described antisocial behavior in male children as resulting from a chain of events leading to these behaviors. These children often had learning difficulties, which led to poor performance at school, problems with peer acceptance, and eventually, frank antisocial behavior. An analogous chain of events may lead to borderline personality disorder: the abusive family coerces the victimized female child to remain isolated and secretive. She has difficulties in school, few trusted companions, and little self-esteem. She leaves home early to escape from the violence but may enter abusive adult relationships. She is at high risk for alcohol abuse. This series of negative environments can be considered the necessary chain of events that leads to the eventual adult outcome of borderline personality disorder.

A review of the scientific evidence indicates that severe and repetitious childhood sexual abuse can constitute an etiological factor leading to borderline psychopathology. Most of the criteria set out for establishing an etiological relation are met to some degree. Childhood sexual abuse is not the only etiological factor in borderline personality disorder, as there is a substantial minority of borderline patients who report no evidence of sexual abuse and another substantial number who report only a single abusive event. Childhood sexual abuse is not a specific etiological factor leading exclusively to the diagnosis of borderline personality disorder, but it is related to certain psychopathological outcomes, such as dissociative features, self-mutilation, and substance abuse. Given the strength of this association, there seems to be no need for further retrospective case-control studies examining the relation between childhood sexual abuse and borderline personality disorder. A careful cohort study following children over time to determine their adult outcomes is needed. However, this is a major undertaking that will require massive resources.

More research is needed on the specific consequences of childhood sexual abuse and its role in predisposing individuals to developing specific disorders in adulthood. Research is also needed on the contributing factors that make childhood sexual abuse so toxic. It appears likely that certain familial factors interact with sexual abuse to explain the eventual risk to the child. Similar findings have been reported in looking at parental loss and adult suicidal behaviors and depression. Parental loss was a risk factor only when preceded by instability and turmoil in the family and when these families were unable to respond constructively and protectively to the crisis (Adam 1994). Further details about the nature of the family environment before, during, and after the abuse are needed.

Value of Psychotherapy for Survivors of Childhood Sexual Abuse

Clinicians have readily adopted the model of the aftereffects of childhood sexual abuse and practice therapeutic approaches to deal with the resolution of these problems. Beutler and Hill (1992), however, have expressed the concern that clinical theory has outstripped the available empirical research. These authors warn that this disparity may lead clinicians to reject empirical research rather than question the validity of their assumptions. In the review described here, we attempt to address this disparity by reviewing the empirical evidence for the effectiveness of psychotherapy for survivors of childhood sexual abuse.

We carried out computerized literature searches of the English literature, using the key words *adult survivors of sexual abuse, psychotherapy, controlled clinical trials, treatment effectiveness evaluation,* and *psychotherapeutic outcomes.* The sources for the search were MEDLINE and Psychological Abstracts or Psych Info. The search covered the period from 1967 to the present and was augmented by the use of key reference papers and discussion with local experts.

Our review was limited to studies evaluating psychotherapeutic interventions; therefore, studies only describing a treatment approach were excluded unless some systematic outcome evaluation was included. Also excluded were studies that dealt with victims of sexual abuse or rape in adulthood.

A search of the literature using the key words *child abuse, sexual,* and *psychotherapy* identified more than 200 references. Nine studies were considered to be relevant to the present discussion. Two of the studies (Feinauer 1989; Perry et al. 1990) were surveys of patients who had undergone psychotherapy to resolve issues related to a history of sexual abuse. Feinauer (1989) found that 20 of 36 women who received therapy believed that they were able to successfully resolve issues related to sexual abuse. Perry et al. (1990) explored the natural history of therapy for psychiatric patients from three diagnostic groups: borderline personality disorder, antisocial personality disorder, and schizotypal personality disorder. The survey revealed that borderline patients believed that it was useful to validate their emotional reactions to their childhood trauma. These patients reported that it was helpful to clarify how their present symptoms were related to the history of childhood trauma. They also valued their therapists' faith that they could and would get better with therapy.

Six of the nine studies were limited to pre- and postevaluations of specific group therapies for adult survivors of childhood sexual abuse (Carver et al. 1989; Davis 1990; Gazan 1986; Jehu 1988; Sultan and Long 1988; Verleur et al. 1986). In the ninth study, Alexander et al. (1989) carried out a randomized control trial of an interpersonal transaction group, a process group, and a "wait-list" control. Sixty-five survivors of incest who had been abused by fathers or stepfathers and were not currently in individual treatment were randomized to the two specific group therapy formats or to the wait-list control group. The study excluded women with serious suicidal ideation (although this was not further defined), psychosis, or severe substance abuse. The primary outcome measures were the patients' symptom levels, as measured by the Beck Depression Inventory (Beck 1978), the Symptom Checklist-90—Revised (SCL90-R; Derogatis 1983), and the Modified Fear Survey (Veronen and Kilpatrick 1980). Social adjustment was measured by the Social Adjustment Scale (Weissman and Bothwell 1976).

The results of the study indicated that there was no significant main effect for treatment type; however, there was a main effect for time, with significant changes in subjects over time in terms of the Beck Depression Inventory, the Modified Fear Survey, and the SCL90-R. There was also a tendency for improvement in all groups, and the interaction of treatment with time was significant. When the groups were compared, it was found that subjects in the two treatment groups showed significant improvement in symptoms of depression after treatment as compared with the wait-list control group. However, the subjects in the process group exhibited greater improvement in their social adjustment, whereas subjects in the wait-list control group deteriorated, and those in the interpersonal transactional group showed a nonsignificant trend toward improvement in role functioning. General measures of distress also showed significant improvement in both treatment groups, whereas the wait-list control subjects exhibited no change in this measure.

A follow-up assessment at 6 months indicated that subjects in both treatment groups not only continued to maintain their improvement but also showed additional improvement over time. The authors believed that this research provided evidence for the efficacy of time-limited group therapies for the treatment of adult survivors of incest. The process group was seen to be particularly effective in enhancing the social adjustment of group participants.

In a related report, Follette et al. (1991) used data from the randomized trial to examine predictors of outcome of the therapeutic intervention. The posttreatment social adjustment score was used as the outcome variable. The variables associated with poor outcome included less education. Subjects who had experienced oral-genital abuse or intercourse did less well than those reporting fondling without penetration. Initial levels of adjustment predicted response to group therapy; higher levels of general distress and depression were associated with poorer outcome. The results also indicated that women who were currently married did less well than those who had no partners. With a stepwise regression, two variables—education and pretherapy Beck Depression Inventory score—were entered into the model to predict outcome. The results of the study indicated that other therapeutic approaches may be needed to maximize therapeutic benefit. Individual therapy, either before or concurrently with group therapy, may be one possible adjunct to the group format used. In addition, marital therapy may be indicated for married survivors of childhood sexual abuse to resolve relationship and sexual dysfunctions related to the aftereffects of the abuse.

Overall, there has been little systematic investigation of psychotherapeutic interventions for adults who survived childhood sexual abuse. Most of the studies reported were pre- and postexaminations without adequate comparison groups or random assignment to treatment. The study by Alexander et al. (1989) stands out from the other studies methodologically and indicates the standard of research that should be striven for in the future.

Eight of the nine studies discuss the benefits of therapy for adult survivors of sexual abuse. The study by Davis (1990) was inconclusive. Alexander et al. (1989) reported benefits from group therapy over the wait-list control group, but there was no particular advantage attributed to the group focused on issues of sexual abuse.

A major finding of the research is that only one study looked at the use of individual therapy in combination with other approaches. The Jehu (1988) study used a cognitive-behavioral approach, but it is very difficult to sort out the specific active ingredients in the study because so many intervention approaches were utilized.

Overall, the studies indicated that there were some specific effects of the treatment interventions. Depression was not changed in three of the studies reported. The randomized control trial (Alexander et al. 1989), however, indicated that the group therapy interventions resulted in a significant decrease in depressive symptoms as compared with the wait-list control group. Three studies showed increased self-esteem after the therapeutic intervention, whereas two others found no change in measures of self-esteem. In terms of general distress measures, the randomized control trial indicated that the group interventions did change the general measure of distress as compared with the wait-list control group. Two other studies found a pre- to postintervention change in general measures of distress. Other significant changes after intervention included improved social adjustment, decreased alienation, improved trust in others, increased sexual awareness, decreased erroneous beliefs, increased sexual responsiveness, and evidence of patient satisfaction after the psychotherapeutic interventions.

It is important to note that a number of aftereffects of childhood sexual abuse have not been used as measures of outcome.

Many adults who experienced sexual abuse in childhood have difficulties in relationships and increased levels of substance abuse, self-mutilation, suicidal ideation and behaviors, dissociative symptoms, and revictimization in adulthood. Future research needs to investigate whether interventions can affect these major behavioral outcomes.

Most of the studies measured outcome only at the end of the treatment intervention. Alexander et al. (1989), however, did measure outcome 6 months after the intervention and indicated that treatment effects continued even after the discontinuation of therapy.

As with other psychotherapy studies, there is some evidence that healthier subjects seem to respond better to treatment (Follette et al. 1991). It is also significant that often the more impaired individuals, that is, those with substance abuse, suicidal ideation, and probably personality disorder diagnoses, were excluded from the trials.

Finally, although the randomized control trial did show benefits resulting from the group interventions, the nonspecific process group seemed to have advantages in terms of psychosocial outcome over the targeted group intervention. It remains unclear as to whether the therapy must be targeted at the experience of childhood trauma.

Implications for Psychotherapy of Patients With Personality Disorders

Our review of the literature indicates several general conclusions that guide our psychotherapeutic work. Survivors of childhood sexual abuse who are diagnosed as adults with personality disorders are likely to have suffered severe and prolonged abuse at the hands of an immediate family member. These patients most often show features of borderline personality disorder, although dissociative disorders can be prominent in survivors of childhood incest (Loewenstein 1993). In therapy, the experience of this abuse must be validated by the therapist. Although individual psychotherapy appears to play an important role in the survivor's recovery, the literature does not suggest that a focus on the traumatic experience is necessary for a successful outcome. In our experience, establishing and maintaining a trusting working alliance is still the primary challenge in working with such patients. Understanding the traumatic antecedents may be most important in terms of providing a framework for the therapist to understand the patient's vexing responses in therapy.

Patients with borderline personality disorder often request individual therapy based on their experience of trauma in childhood. These patients find individual therapy much more satisfying than group therapy. They have difficulty giving up being the focus of attention and have a reluctance to participate in groups. Individual therapy for borderline patients may be needed to "break the silence" surrounding their history of sexual abuse. Often the repressed material will emerge in the context of a trusting relationship. Judith Herman, in her excellent book *Trauma and Recovery* (Herman 1992), indicated that the patient must first establish a safe environment for herself or himself before dealing with the traumatic history. Establishing personal safety may come through building the patient's ego strengths before working through the traumatic history (Gunderson and Chu 1993; Herman 1992). Safety in the therapy relationship will be encouraged when the patient feels that the experience and pain from the childhood abuse have been accepted and understood by the therapist (Gunderson and Chu 1993). For many of these patients, a sense of personal safety must first be established by assisting them in changing their living environments. The therapist may have to address those current relationships of the patient that make the patient unsafe. In one case, a female patient with a history of abuse felt unable even to walk the halls in the hospital or to attend group sessions when men were present. She experienced terror at night because of the very real fear that a man might enter her hospital room at night. The therapist may have to attend to the patient's abuse of substances or of self as the initial interventions to ensure the patient's safety.

Safety may be defined in a very personal way:

Case 1

Mr. A, a 28-year-old gay man, presented to therapy with frequent, almost daily, urges to self-mutilate. Several times a month, he would cut himself on various parts of his body. He reported an addicting sense of relief when he watched blood ooze from his wounds. However, he kept these urges and behaviors a total secret. Even his current partner had no knowledge of his self-mutilation.

Mr. A's history revealed a very turbulent childhood, and he acknowledged that "there is a high probability" that he had been sexually abused. His mother had taken up with a series of alcoholic and abusive men. A previous therapist had suggested to Mr. A that his self-abuse might be related to a history of childhood sexual abuse. Despite the fact that he felt a great desperation to change his life and put an end to his "secret," Mr. A did not wish to explore this issue in therapy. He accepted the explanation that he had to feel safe before he could proceed with making further changes in his life.

Over the next few weeks, he came to understand that moving back to his hometown, closer to his ailing mother, would give him a feeling of greater safety. With a well-formulated plan, he moved to his hometown as the first step toward making changes.

Group therapy may have a role in counteracting the "myth of silence" that the perpetrator and the family forced or fostered in the sexually abused patient. Individual therapy may be used to prepare for the patient's involvement in a group for survivors of childhood sexual abuse.

Research performed to date has not studied samples of patients with both personality disorders and a history of childhood sexual abuse, nor has it addressed outcomes relevant to this population of patients. Future research will have to examine changes in level of substance abuse, self-mutilation, suicidal behaviors, other acts of impulsivity, and victimization in other relationships as important outcomes.

Current theoretical models of the treatment of childhood sexual abuse may not be entirely appropriate for patients with personality disorders. Gunderson and Chu (1993) discussed methods of incorporating the trauma history into the therapy of patients with borderline personality disorder. Maintenance of the therapeutic distance in the relationship and dealing with countertransference remain as the primary challenges with patients who have borderline personality disorder. Gabbard and Wilkinson (1994) have authored a book providing many insights into handling therapists' countertransferential responses.

The models of therapy of survivors may need to be modified in other ways as well. For example, confrontation of the perpetrator is considered an important step to end the victimization that the patient has suffered. Although this step may be an important one to empower the patient, it may be inappropriate for a patient with a diagnosis of personality disorder. Often the perpetrators, for example, the fathers, are severely disordered themselves. They often have major personality disorders or substance abuse problems that may make such a confrontation of little therapeutic benefit and may even put the patient at physical risk.

In our experience, the history of abuse does not become a focus at a specific time in therapy. A certain level of trust must first be established before the issue is discussed. Our initial stance, however, is to indicate to the patient that his or her recollections of the experience are believed and that his or her pain and suffering are validated. Throughout the therapy, which may be several years in duration, we attempt to indicate a perpetual acceptance of the need to discuss the trauma. This allows the patient to address this issue at various times during the course of therapy. Initial validation and continuing acceptance enable the issues to come up over time within the context of a trusting patient-therapist relationship.

We have utilized the victimization syndrome, as outlined by McCarthy (1990), to indicate how the traumatic history affects the patient's current life. McCarthy describes three levels of victimization: the first relates to the actual sexual incidents themselves, the second concerns how the sexual incidents are revealed and dealt with, and the third entails the patient's adopting the lifelong label of "victim." Typically, the abused borderline patient has a history of experiencing one traumatic environment after another—for example, an incestuous family, an unrewarding school life, and a series of traumatizing relationships. Therapists must guard against the therapy's becoming another traumatic experience and must attend carefully to the boundaries of the patient-therapist relationship. The victimized borderline patient can appear very helpless and may make escalating demands on the therapist. Because of the therapist's countertransference rescue fantasies, the therapist may slowly relax his or her established boundaries by extending sessions, taking telephone calls at home at any hour, or offering physical closeness. Patients can become mired in the traumatic experience, losing sight of their current life and relationships. These patients are "almost fixated on retrieving and exploring the traumatic memories" (Gunderson and Chu 1993, p. 77).

Case 2

Ms. B had made significant gains in resolving her abusive past. She was extremely motivated to recall further events from her past, including "some happy memories." Her energies were taken up with trying to stimulate recall of certain past events. Nonetheless, her feelings of helplessness and anger only seemed to intensify. As her distress approached crisis proportions, she finally made mention of her teenaged son, who had moved back into her apartment over the last few weeks. He had quickly turned Ms. B's life "upside down" and was showing total disregard for "the house rules." Ms. B was confronted with her need to end the current victimization and to not lose sight of the present because of the past.

This problem can be overcome by encouraging the patient to focus on the present and how his or her identity can be shifted from that of a victim to that of a survivor.

It is difficult to know whether to focus on the abuse experience or the symptoms that may be a result of it. We believe that it is important to make the connection between the abuse experience and the current symptoms. As Perry et al. (1990) have pointed out, this knowledge seems important to patients and helps them come to some understanding of themselves. However, if the symptoms manifest to a degree where they jeopardize the patient's safety or have an impact on establishing a working therapeutic relationship, then they must be dealt with as a first priority.

Conclusion

Childhood sexual abuse predisposes the victim to significant difficulties in adulthood, and survivors of severe and repetitious abuse may show borderline psychopathology. As Paris and Zweig-Frank (1992) pointed out, we must clarify the exact nature of the etiological role of childhood sexual abuse so that better models and more specific therapies can be developed. We also must be able to target our psychotherapeutic interventions to the needs of the particular patient. For example, a married woman with a history of childhood sexual abuse may be helped more by couple therapy, whereas individual therapy may place stress on the marital relationship. Individual therapy may assist the woman to personally resolve the trauma, but it will not address the couple's level of intimacy and sexual functioning.

The therapist's understanding of the traumatic experience is crucial to working with survivors of sexual abuse, but no model of therapy can be a panacea for these patients. Although much remains to be learned, psychotherapy for patients with a history of childhood sexual abuse appears to be a humane way to help these patients achieve improved health.

References

Adam KS: Suicidal behaviour and attachment: a developmental model, in Attachment in Adults: Theory, Life Span Development and Treatment Issues. Edited by Sperling MB, Berman WH. New York, Guilford, 1994, pp 275–298

Alexander PC, Neimeyer RA, Folette VM, et al: A comparison of group treatments of women sexually abused as children. J Consult Clin Psychol 57:479–483, 1989

Beck AT: Depression Inventory. Philadelphia, PA, Philadelphia Center for Cognitive Therapy, 1978

Beutler LE, Hill CE: Process and outcome research in the treatment of adult victims of childhood sexual abuse: methodological issues. J Consult Clin Psychol 60:204–212, 1992

Briere J, Runtz M: The long-term effects of sexual abuse: a review and synthesis. New Dir Ment Health Serv 51:3–13, 1991

Brown GR, Anderson B: Psychiatric morbidity in adult inpatients with histories of sexual and physical abuse. Am J Psychiatry 148:55–61, 1991

Browne A, Finkelhor D: Impact of sexual abuse: a review of the research. Psychol Bull 99:66–77, 1986

Bryer JB, Nelson BA, Miller JB, et al: Childhood sexual and physical abuse as factors in adult psychiatric illness. Am J Psychiatry 144:1426–1430, 1987

Carver CM, Stalker C, Stewart E, et al: The impact of group therapy for adult survivors of childhood sexual abuse. Can J Psychiatry 34:753–758, 1989

Davis KR: Emotional and interpersonal changes that occur during the course of time-limited, structured group treatment for adult survivors of childhood sexual abuse. Dissertation Abstracts International 50(8):3688-B, 1990

Derogatis L: SCL-90-R Manual II. Towson, MD, Clinical Psychometric Research, 1983

Feinauer LL: Relationship of treatment to adjustment in women sexually abused as children. American Journal of Family Therapy 17:326–334, 1989

Follette VM, Alexander PC, Folette WC: Individual predictors of outcome in group treatment for incest survivors. J Consult Clin Psychol 59:150–155, 1991

Gabbard GO, Wilkinson SM: Management of Countertransference With Borderline Patients. Washington, DC, American Psychiatric Press, 1994

Gazan M: An evaluation of a treatment package designed for women with a history of sexual victimization in childhood and sexual dysfunctions in adulthood. Canadian Journal of Community Mental Health 5:85–102, 1986

Gunderson J, Chu JA: Treatment implications of past trauma in borderline personality disorder. Harvard Review of Psychiatry 1:75–81, 1993

Herman JL: Trauma and Recovery. New York, Basic Books, 1992

Herman JL, Schatzow E: Recovery and verification of memories of childhood sexual trauma. Psychoanalytic Psychology 4:1–14, 1987

Herman JL, Perry JC, van der Kolk B: Childhood trauma in borderline personality disorder. Am J Psychiatry 146:490–495, 1989

Jehu D: Beyond Sexual Abuse: Therapy With Women Who Were Childhood Victims. Chichester, Great Britain, Wiley, 1988

Links PS, van Reekum R: Childhood sexual abuse, parental impairment and the development of borderline personality disorder. Can J Psychiatry 38:472–474, 1993

Links PS, Steiner M, Offord D, et al: Characteristics of borderline personality disorder: a Canadian study. Can J Psychiatry 33:336–340, 1988

Links PS, Boiago I, Huxley G, et al: Sexual abuse and biparental failure as etiologic models in borderline personality disorder, in Family Environment and Borderline Personality Disorder. Edited by Links PS. Washington, DC, American Psychiatric Press, 1990, pp 105–120

Loewenstein RJ: Aspects of the treatment of dissociative disorders in survivors of incest, in Treatment of Adult Survivors of Incest. Edited by Paddison PL. Washington, DC, American Psychiatric Press, 1993, pp 77–99

Ludolph PS, Westen D, Misle B, et al: The borderline diagnosis in adolescents: symptoms and developmental history. Am J Psychiatry 147:470–476, 1990

McCarthy BW: Treating sexual dysfunction associated with prior sexual trauma. J Sex Marital Ther 16:142–146, 1990

Ogata SN, Silk KR, Goodrich S, et al: Childhood sexual and physical abuse in adult patients with borderline personality disorder. Am J Psychiatry 147:1008–1013, 1990

Paris J, Zweig-Frank H: A critical review of the role of childhood sexual abuse in the etiology of borderline personality disorder. Can J Psychiatry 37:125–128, 1992

Paris J, Zweig-Frank H, Guzder J: Psychological risk factors for borderline personality disorder in female patients. Compr Psychiatry 35:301–305, 1994

Perry JC, Herman JL: Trauma and defense in the etiology of borderline personality disorder, in Borderline Personality Disorder: Etiology and Treatment. Edited by Paris J. Washington, DC, American Psychiatric Press, 1993, pp 123–139

Perry JC, Herman JL, van der Kolk BA, et al: Psychotherapy and psychological trauma in borderline personality disorder. Psychiatric Annals 20:33–43, 1990

Robins LN, Schoenberg SP, Holmes SJ, et al: Early home environment and retrospective recall: a test for concordance between siblings with and without psychiatric disorders. Am J Orthopsychiatry 55:27–41, 1985

Russell D: The Secret Trauma: Incest in the Lives of Girls and Women. New York, Basic Books, 1986

Rutter M, Giller H: Juvenile Delinquency: Trends and Perspectives. New York, Guilford, 1984

Stone MH, Kahn E, Flye B: Psychiatrically ill relatives of borderline patients: a family study. Psychiatr Q 53:71–84, 1981

Sultan FE, Long GT: Treatment of the sexually/physically abused female inmate: evaluation of an intensive short-term intervention program. Journal of Offender Counselling Services and Rehabilitation 12:131–143, 1988

Verleur D, Hughes RE, Dobkin de Rios M: Enhancement of self-esteem among female adolescent incest victims: a controlled comparison. Adolescence 21:843–854, 1986

Veronen LJ, Kilpatrick DG: Reported fears of rape victims: a preliminary investigation. Behav Modif 4:383–396, 1980

Weissman MM, Bothwell S: Assessment of social adjustment by patient self-report. Arch Gen Psychiatry 33:111–115, 1976

Westen D, Ludolph P, Misle B, et al: Physical and sexual abuse in adolescent girls with borderline personality disorder. Am J Orthopsychiatry 60:55–66, 1990

Zanarini MC, Gunderson JG, Marino MF: Childhood experiences of borderline patients. Compr Psychiatry 30:18–25, 1989

Zanarini M, Dubo ED, Lewis RE, et al: The relationship between sexual abuse and borderline personality disorder. Paper presented at the annual meeting of the American Psychiatric Association, San Francisco, CA, May 1993

Zweig-Frank H, Paris J, Guzder J: Psychological risk factors for dissociation and self-mutilation in female patients with borderline personality disorder. Can J Psychiatry 39:259–264, 1994

CHAPTER 10

Helping the Family: A Framework for Intervention

M. Janice E. Mitton, B.A., R.N., M.H.Sc.
Paul S. Links, M.D., M.Sc., F.R.C.P.C.

*D*rawing on the literature, on other clinicians working in this area, and on clinical experience, in this chapter we review and expand on current knowledge (both clinical/descriptive and empirical) about the needs of family members of adults with personality disorders. A framework for providing support and education to these families is explored and summarized. Available resources are listed, and a brief description of written materials and services is provided.

The overall goals of this chapter are

- To provide an overview of current knowledge about the effect of personality disorder on the family
- To educate clinicians about the needs of family members of individuals with personality disorders
- To provide a flexible, adaptable framework within which clinicians may assist these family members

Throughout this chapter, individuals with personality disorders or with troublesome traits of personality disorder are referred to as *patients*. The term *family* refers to extended family members or friends who are affected by the patient's personality style and who are potential sources of support for the patient.

According to the distinction described by Oldham and Morris (1990), personality *style* refers to common, nonpathological traits and attitudes that make each individual unique and characterize one's manner of relating to the world. Personality *disorder* refers to constellations of extremes of these normal traits and attitudes (Oldham and Morris 1990). In addition, the view is taken that personality disorder constitutes a form of serious mental illness that jeopardizes the patient's ability to be fully functional across many areas of his or her life.

Although certain personality disorders, such as borderline, narcissistic, and antisocial personality disorders, have had broad and extensive coverage in the clinical and research literature, there is little information about the functioning of individuals with these or other personality disorders in close, personal relationships. One need only review the descriptions and core criteria for personality disorders in DSM-IV (American Psychiatric Association 1994), however, to understand that one of the basic features of these individuals is severe interpersonal dysfunction. For example, contained in its overview of personality disorders, it is noted in DSM-IV that the "behaviors or traits cause significant impairment in social . . . functioning" (American Psychiatric Association 1994, p. 630). This is described as a core feature for any personality disorder; specific criteria are noted in the more extensive descriptions provided for each personality disorder (see Chapter 2 for DSM-IV criteria for each personality disorder).

In addition, the clinical literature offers guidelines and suggestions to clinicians in treating and managing the therapeutic relationship with individuals with various personality disorders (Adler 1989; Alden 1989; Deltito and Perugi 1986; Deltito and Stam 1989; DuBrul 1989; Goulet 1988; Heimberg and Barlow 1991; Kaplan 1986; Masterson 1990; Mattick and Newman 1991; McCann 1988; Messer 1985; Oldham 1988; Piccinino 1990; Renneberg et al. 1990; Royal Australian and New Zealand College of Psychiatrists 1991; S. C. Schulz et al. 1988; Wells et al. 1990). A limited amount of literature exists on working with couples in which one partner has a personality disorder (Chernen and Friedman 1993; Lachkar 1986; Slavik et al. 1992). For the most part, however, little attention has been paid to assisting the parents, siblings, spouses, children, and other family members of patients with personality disorders in managing their close relationships with the patient or to considering the family's involvement in the ongoing treatment plan.

Despite family-oriented care being widely acclaimed in health care, the issue of helping families cope with a member who has been diagnosed with a personality disorder has received little attention (Hartman and Boerger 1989). The research literature has amply documented that knowledge about a mental illness leads to more positive patterns of interaction and communication on the part of the relatives of an ill family member and that this in turn can have a positive impact on prognosis (Berkowitz et al. 1984; Brown et al. 1972).

Background

It is likely that family members of patients with personality disorders know little about the manifestations, course, treatment, or outcome of these illnesses. Yet family members are often the "front line workers" who regularly face, and may be deeply and personally affected by, the patient's confusing, perplexing, annoying, inconvenient, or frightening behaviors. The following three case examples illustrate some of the difficulties that may bring the family members of an individual with a personality disorder to a clinician's attention:

Case 1

Ms. A has requested a referral for marital counseling. As she describes her situation, the antisocial characteristics of her spouse become apparent. She has just reconciled with her husband of 2 years after their third brief separation. She has now given him an ultimatum: either he finds a job he can keep and stops running to his parents every time he needs bailing out financially, or she will end the marriage. Her husband's erratic employment record has resulted in his quitting jobs because of boredom or, more typically, in his being fired after verbal and physical conflicts with supervisors and co-workers. Ms. A also reports that he has struck her and her 6-year-old daughter on several occasions, at times resulting in bruising. Adding to her frustration is his failure to see any point of view but his own.

Case 2

Mr. B presents to his family physician with chronic, stress-related headaches that have not responded to prescribed medications. His presentation is compatible with a diagnosis of paranoid personality disorder. He has felt increasing pressures and anxiety at work in the past several months. With this has come an exaggeration of his usual suspiciousness and mistrust of others, his irrational feelings of jealousy toward his wife, and his tendency to respond with verbal and physical aggression to what he perceives to be slights and insults. Although he states that he is uncomfortable divulging all of this personal information, even to his physician, he nevertheless shows some insight into his problems and fears their effects on his marriage. Mr. B would like to understand himself better and wonders whether couple counseling would be of benefit to him and his wife.

Case 3

Mr. C is once again seeking a referral for psychotherapy. His mother (who is well known to the local psychiatric service as having borderline personality disorder) has been readmitted for depression and suicidal threats. Mr. C is fed up with her "blackmailing behavior" and is tired of serving as her "emotional soother." He also admits that his own attempts to calm his nerves with alcohol and street drugs may be getting out of hand.

The dilemmas of these family members may be compounded when the health care professionals from whom they seek assistance face their own uncertain knowledge (and, possibly, inexperience) in recognizing, understanding, managing, and treating a patient with a personality disorder. Indeed, it was only in 1980 that the diagnoses of personality disorders were given more prominence by placing them on a separate Axis in DSM-III (American Psychiatric Association 1980). The latest version, DSM-IV, was published in 1994. With these changes, and the current uncertainty even among experts in personality disorders about how best to categorize these disorders, it is not surprising that health care professionals have been reluctant to speak freely and openly about the "problem," "condition," or "illness" to patients who may have a personality disorder or to their relatives.

The present situation of protecting ourselves, our patients, and our patients' families is not unlike the approach taken to schizophrenia more than two decades ago. At that time, health care professionals often avoided open discussions about the illness, even after they were certain of the diagnosis. Families were not usually included in treatment planning, yet many patients were discharged home to the family's care. In addition, it was not unusual for family members, especially parents, to receive direct or covert messages that they either were the cause of or had made major contributions to the patient's becoming ill. Since that time, research on the family's involvement in the schizophrenic patient's treatment and ongoing care has led to numerous articles, books, support groups, and educational programs that have assisted and enabled families to be actively and positively involved in the lives and holistic treatment of their affected relative. Our clinical and research work has led us to conclude that the families of patients with personality disorders would benefit from a similar attitude and an approach aimed at educating and supporting them in their relationships with their affected family member.

Role of the Modern Family and Its Response to Illness

Because of cultural norms that stress independence and privacy, the nuclear family represents the norm in modern North American society. Given this relative isolation, each relationship within the family takes on critical importance for the provision of stability to family members. This, and the fairly impersonal characteristics of social relationships outside the family, provides for uniquely intense and highly emotional ties among family members (Bell and Vogel 1968). Typically, parents provide a crucial caregiving role for children, and this role often extends to adult family members who need special support (Spaniol et al. 1992).

With the continuing trend toward deinstitutionalization of psychiatrically ill or troubled patients and the reality of shrinking health care dollars, families are increasingly being asked to fill in the gaps of what must seem to be an ever-narrowing range of services. Families do not readily choose this role, and furthermore, they often lack the knowledge, skills, and external support systems required to provide specialized care (Spaniol et al. 1992).

Illness, especially a chronic illness, and including one with an unpredictable pattern of relapse or exacerbation, often leads to imbalances within the arranged roles and responsibilities of family members.

For example, on several occasions, Mr. C (Case 3) has found himself performing caretaking tasks with or for his mother. He has been called by his mother's therapist for input on the mother's current mental status, has physically restrained his mother when she was refusing admission to the hospital, and is perpetually cautious in his expectations for a more positive relationship with her. He finds it bewildering that, although his mother seems to get much worse during her hospitalizations, staff seem anxious to discharge her. Only on one occasion has anyone sat down with the two of them to offer assistance in diffusing the widening gulf of anger and pain between them. Mr. C still does not understand "what's wrong with her."

Because by its very nature a personality disorder is characterized as a lifelong illness that is usually apparent by adolescence, the family's attitude toward and involvement with the patient will depend, in part, on the length of time they have been attempting to cope with the patient's behaviors, their success in doing so, and whether they perceive themselves to have a supportive network for their efforts.

To cite another example, although Ms. A (Case 1) expresses a desire to stay in her marriage, her husband's actions are slowly eroding her will to do so and are also aggravating her ability to cope with her current level of stress. His inability to contribute financially to the family has resulted in four moves in the past 2 years. Ms. A's daughter has been in as many schools and is beginning to display a withdrawn, sad mood. Ms. A cannot turn to her own family for support because they unsympathetically tell her to leave her husband and do not wish to be associated with him themselves.

Research has consistently found that mental illness produces considerable burdens for family members and results in significant impairment, particularly in the areas of role functioning and communication. In a study of the family members of patients who had either borderline or schizotypal personality disorder, the burden experienced by the family was slightly greater than those of the families of patients with severe physical illnesses but less than those of families with a member who had schizophrenia. Antisocial acts by the patient, financial strain, dependency of the patient, and the patient's inability to remain employed were rated as particularly burdensome (P. M. Schulz et al. 1985).

The family of a patient with psychiatric difficulties may cycle regularly through hope and despair because of the lack of clarity around the process and outcome of the illness. This can produce a delayed grief reaction as the family continues to hold out hope that the ill relative will eventually return to or attain normal functioning (Miller et al. 1990; Spaniol et al. 1992; Tonge et al. 1975).

The family's level of distress also depends on the responsibility that they bear for direct or indirect care of the patient and the amount and kind of assistance available from outside sources (Hatfield and LeFley 1987). It has been observed, for example, that the families of mentally ill individuals in developing countries are better able to tolerate their affected relative's aberrant behavior, partially as a result of extended kinship networks that provide a large support system, dilute highly charged emotional relationships, and extend a sense of genuine concern (LeFley 1987). The family's responses to the patient may be further exacerbated when the patient lives with the family (Maurin and Boyd 1990).

Another powerful factor affecting the level of distress experienced by the family with an ill member, as well as their response to him or her, is the meaning that a society assigns to an illness. In North American culture, self-reliance is valued and supported by belief in an "internal locus of control"; that is, the individual is responsible and accountable for his or her feelings, actions, and destiny. The individual with a personality disorder typically expresses symptoms of the illness through behavior. Psychological problems that cannot be attributed to known external causes, such as genetic disorders, viral illness, or trauma, are attributed to patients themselves and/or to their families. This situation can make it difficult for family members to feel or express support for and understanding of the patient. In addition, it may be equally difficult for them to seek or receive support and understanding from the outside world.

In addition to programs that educate and teach coping skills, social support has proved to be a significant mediator of the burdens of families of patients with a psychiatric illness (Hatfield and LeFley 1987; Mannion et al. 1994; Melges and Swartz 1989;

Ryglewicz 1991; Spaniol et al. 1992). In the absence of such formal programs or groups to provide these services to and support family members of individuals with personality disorders, we propose in this chapter a modified version of such a program that could be delivered by a primary caregiver involved with the family.

Current State of Knowledge

In a study that measured the impact of borderline and schizotypal personality disorder pathology on patients and their families, P. M. Schulz et al. (1985) measured families' burdens, as well as their attitudes and knowledge about the illness. These authors found that families had to deal with many of the same issues found in the families of patients with chronic mental or physical disorders. These issues included considerable burden on the family unit, difficulty dealing with troublesome symptoms and behaviors, chronic economic problems, and stress. Patients and their families often knew little about the disorders, and family members felt excluded from the treatment process. In their own work, the authors found that discussions with patients and relatives about the presentation of the disorders, their possible relation to other psychiatric disorders, and the results of treatment trials were gratefully accepted (P. M. Schulz et al. 1985).

Melges and Swartz (1989) recognized that family members of borderline patients were mystified and exhausted by aspects of their relative's illness. They found that bringing the family together to discuss their problems and providing a psychoeducational approach served as the first step toward improving family relationships.

Clinicians currently working with individuals with personality disorders acknowledge that there is no empirical evidence and little clinical experience to support the benefits of working with the family members of these individuals (J. Paris, B. Pfohl, and J. Kreisman, personal communication, July 1993). Silk (K. Silk, personal communication, November 1993) emphasizes the following points when working with the families of patients with borderline personality disorder:

- **Education:** The family needs to be educated that the long-term outcome (i.e., 7–15 years) is good for most borderline patients to return to normal functioning. Patients and their families often benefit from receiving recommended reading lists to increase their understanding of personality disorders and to facilitate the development of constructive coping strategies.
- **Alliance:** An alliance needs to be established with the family so that they can understand the value and limitations of therapy. Jones (1987) also attends to forming an alliance with the family when working with borderline, narcissistic individuals in order to utilize the family's influence in the treatment of these difficult patients.
- **Support:** The family needs support (as opposed to criticism) and constructive options to deal with the patient's behaviors. With a good working alliance, the family will reciprocate by supporting the therapist's interventions.

Kreisman and colleagues at St. John's Mercy Medical Center, Bethesda, Maryland, have found that an educational format that defines and explains troublesome behaviors as characteristic of the presentation of a patient with a personality disorder is helpful to family members. Specific Axis II diagnoses, however, are named directly or acknowledged as being associated with a particular personality disorder only if the family specifically asks for this information (J. Kreisman, personal communication, July 1993). In our clinical experience, outpatients with personality disorders who had extensive histories of emotional or psychiatric difficulties; social, interpersonal, and occupational dysfunction; contacts with the medical system; and psychiatric treatment have generally responded favorably to hearing the personality disorder named.

The St. John's Mercy Medical Center clinic also offers a monthly 2-hour open support group for patients and their families. During the first hour, an educational format is employed, and different speakers address particular areas of concern, such as managing suicidal gestures or threats. In the second hour, patients and families are separated into two groups led by staff members, who may then discuss individual responses or questions related to the content of the presentation. A problem-oriented approach is then used to deal with individual experiences related to the topic area under discussion. This also gives family members an opportunity to discuss more sensitive issues without the patient's being present and to benefit from the input and support of peers. As yet, there has been no follow-up of clinic patients and their families in order to evaluate the effectiveness of these interventions.

Family involvement during long-term inpatient hospitalization can benefit the family by validating the feelings of all family members and quelling the blaming response for the patient's illness. At the Psychotherapy Treatment Unit in Whitby Psychiatric Hospital, Whitby, Ontario, Canada, the average length of stay is 12–15 months. Most of the patients have a diagnosis of borderline personality disorder and have childhood histories of sexual abuse. Approximately 50%–60% of patients' families are involved in their treatment, usually 4–5 months into the hospitalization, after the patient is stabilized and amenable to family work. The average number of family sessions is flexible, although in the experience of staff, the sessions typically number three to four. The sessions may take a number of formats, from open discussion with the entire family about the rationale for the patient's hospitalization, to eventual disclosure of abuse and management of its aftereffects. The Whitby Psychotherapy Treatment Unit also provides couple sessions for patients and their spouses. This also comes later in the patient's stay, the emphasis initially being on support and inclusion of the partner, followed by an educational approach (M. Brennan, personal communication, July 1993).

In our own clinical and research work with individuals with personality disorders (described further later in this chapter), we have observed that family members have unmet needs for education, knowledge, and support concerning their family member with personality disorder or traits of personality disorder. A sample of 15 family members of 10 individuals with personality disorders (who had been referred to our clinic, which specializes in the assessment and management of outpatients with personality disorders) completed a self-report questionnaire that assessed their needs in relation to the patient. All respondents indicated a desire for information related to the cause and future course of their relative's illness. Interest was also shown for general information about the condition (80% positive response rate) and treatment (93%), as well as the risk to other family members for developing the condition (67%).

More than half of the respondents indicated a need for professional assistance for themselves regarding the patient (67%), as well an interest in the development of a community support group (60%). Relatives rated previous care received by the patient as poor (43% of responses), and only 9% indicated satisfaction with information received from health care providers regarding their relative with personality disorder.

Our data also suggested the need by family members for education about personality disorders. Just over half of the respondents (53%) believed their family member to have a personality disorder. (This finding may be inflated, given the name of our team, the "Personality Investigation Team.") Although only 66% of the family members believed their ill relative to have a psychiatric disorder, 80% nevertheless chose depression as the category of illness (Mitton et al. 1993).

These observations and our review of current knowledge in the area have resulted in the development of a model for intervention with the family members of individuals with personality disorders. The model is based on existing and successful models reported in the research and clinical literature for use with the families of patients who have been diagnosed with other major psychiatric illnesses, such as schizophrenia.

Nature Versus Nurture

Although some studies have found a positive link between environment (particularly negative experiences during childhood) and the development of personality disorder, to date there are no hard data to support environmental influences as specific causal factors. Current thinking supports the view of an interactive model in which personality results from the interplay between an individual's unique genetic makeup and the environment of his or her family of origin. This is then further reinforced by life experiences and the larger environment—for example, trauma, culture, peer group, and social and world events (Oldham and Morris 1990; Waldinger 1984). (Chapter 9 presents a discussion on the relation between childhood sexual abuse and borderline personality disorder.) These interactive forces continue throughout a person's lifetime, so that problematic family relationships may predispose, facilitate, or perpetuate the emergence or expression of personality disorder, and vice versa.

In Case 3, for example, Mr. C's mother had suffered extreme physical abuse from her alcoholic father during childhood. This led her to leave home as a teenager. She married a drug addict at age 19, and this was also an abusive relationship, as were several later ones. Inadequate parenting and unresolved issues from her childhood not only interfered with her ability to meet her own needs and to form healthy relationships but also disabled her as a parent.

The above observations regarding nature versus nurture are not meant to exonerate the role of noxious early family or extrafamilial environments in which obvious instances of abuse clearly continue to have a large effect on the patient's difficulties and expression of illness. Indeed, when personality disorder is suspected, the clinician must attempt to take a careful and complete history of past and present abuses and trauma. In the presence of continuing severe abuse, in whatever form, it is necessary to counsel and support the patient or family member in establishing a safe environment, that is, physical distance or separation from the perpetrator. It will then be necessary to determine whether the victim or survivor wishes to maintain contact with the perpetrator(s). A supportive, empathic, nonconfrontational stance is helpful in assisting the patient in dealing further with the impact of abuse on his or her current life situation. The resources offered should include the choice of therapeutic interventions beyond the clinician's scope or availability, such as support groups, psychotherapy, and other therapies.

When a history of abuse has been disclosed and a member of the nuclear family has been identified as the perpetrator, it may help the clinician to note that abusive parents are often the products of very troubled family backgrounds themselves. The additional challenge is then to privately view them with the same level of compassion that is directed toward the patient. Although each party may feel the urge to blame the other for his or her current difficulties, they both need assistance in accepting responsibility for their individual roles in the present relationship. This may be the first step in allowing change to occur (Cauwels 1992).

An Interactive Framework for Intervention

The framework presented here, intended for work with the families of individuals with personality disorders, is based on existing clinical experience and knowledge. It is meant to be used in a dynamic manner in which it is recognized that families operate as systems within other systems. Key points from the framework appear throughout the text in italics as they are explained and expanded on.

Goal

The overall goal of working with the families of patients with personality disorders is *to engage the family; the patient, where indicated; and the clinician in collaborative and therapeutic interactions.* This is an ongoing, dynamic process that will be continually shaped by the interactive forces that have an effect on all participants.

Challenges and Implementation

One of the major challenges to reaching this goal is *recognizing and understanding the behaviors, attitudes, and feelings* that each participant, that is, the *clinician,* the *family,* and the *patient,* brings to the collaborative process. As *clinicians,* we must take care that our *attitudes* and expressed beliefs do not communicate to the family that we hold them responsible for causing the patient's illness or that we believe that their interactions might be perpetuating it. This will only further burden the family and will alienate them from a potential source of support and education.

Conversely, concentrating too heavily on an illness model, that is, on the idea that the patient has an illness, disease, or mental condition, may be misinterpreted as a covert message that the patient is not responsible for his or her behavior or that the situation is hopeless. For example, further information obtained in Case 3 (Mr. C) indicated that his mother had an intolerance for being alone, expressed wildly vacillating opinions of her friends and family members, and had frequent, severe mood changes, all of which supported a diagnosis of borderline personality disorder. Although this is a very serious disorder and one that is particularly draining on family members, Mr. C needs reassurance that his own actions and response to his mother do not create or exacerbate her symptoms. Furthermore, although his mother's expression of her illness is beyond his control, Mr. C may be able to reduce its effects on himself through education about and training in more healthy patterns of responding to her verbal and physical communications.

The *feelings, beliefs,* and *attitudes* of *family* members and their interactions with the patient are influenced by earlier contacts with the health care system. If they have previously sought assistance in dealing with their relative with a personality disorder, the family may present as frustrated, skeptical, and distrustful because of past encounters with the medical system or health care providers. It is very likely that, at the least, they have been given contradictory information and advice. The norm is for major psychiatric disturbances, such as depression, anxiety disorders, and substance abuse or dependence, to coexist with personality disorder and to be the target(s) for attention and treatment. In addition, more than one personality disorder is almost invariably present. It is quite possible that the term *personality disorder* has never been mentioned by health care providers and that it is a new concept for both the patient and family.

In addition, if the patient has had a long history of contacts with the mental health system, the family may also be feeling the social stigma and ostracization that too often accompany mental illness. This in itself can present a barrier to collaboration with the clinician. An empathic relationship with a neutral caregiver may be the first step to healing past and present wounds.

Initially, a professional, nonaffective stance and the (apparently simple) art of listening to the family's presentation of the problem(s) may begin the process of diffusing the situation and providing a sense of relief and hope. The initial assessment will begin the process of *creating a positive environment* between the family and the clinician, which will lead to facilitating a positive environment between the family and the patient. A problem-solving approach should be taken with the family and/or the patient. The goal is to hear from each member his or her statement or understanding of the problem and its past and present effects on an immediate, short-term, and long-term basis. This is a good first step in *collaborative interaction.* From this information, the clinician should also be able to extrapolate the troublesome behaviors of the patient (which may also serve in diagnosing the predominant personality style) and in identifying the resultant transactional problems facing the family system (Wrate et al. 1987).

To illustrate this point, Mr. B and his wife (Case 2) were seen together and he reviewed, with the clinician's assistance, the difficulties he was having in controlling his fears and beliefs about the intent of others' actions and communications. His wife was very supportive and was able to provide further evidence of how Mr. B looked for hidden motives and was quick to accuse or counterattack, thus confirming the clinician's diagnosis of paranoid personality disorder. Mr. B's wife acknowledged that these characteristics had become more troublesome in the past several months as the pressures of his job increased. Whereas previously she had been able to talk him through his misperceptions, she herself had come under attack from him lately; for instance, he had taken to interrogating her about her whereabouts, which she interpreted as a form of surveillance.

At this point in treatment, the process of *educating* the family could begin with a discussion of the general characteristics of personality disorders, as well as the fact that they are not under the patient's immediate control. These characteristics include

- Long-standing, rigid, inflexible patterns of behavior in response to situations and people, which are especially apparent during times of stress and are less amenable to change than are episodic conditions, such as depression
- Lack of insight or the inability to understand that a problem exists and, often, lack of empathy, so that there is little appreciation for the effects of the behaviors on others
- Disability in relating to others that is generally serious and pervasive, though not always incapacitating
- Ability to elicit an often strong and unconscious emotional response from others, ranging from despair to anger

The family should also understand that the persistent dysfunctional beliefs of an individual with a personality disorder are built into his or her normal way of perceiving the world. Therefore, changing these beliefs, or at least assisting the patient in managing his or her response to situations and to others because of them, will require considerable time and effort (Beck and Freeman 1990).

The family should also be provided with information on each of the personality disorders. An excellent resource for the lay person is *Personality Self-Portrait* (Oldham and Morris 1990). This book provides a method for self-assessment in the area of personality. It contains practical suggestions for the constructive utilization of one's own traits and those of others, as well as appropriate responses to troublesome traits. (See the list of resources at the end of this chapter.)

Another useful approach to understanding personality disorders is outlined in *Cognitive Therapy of Personality Disorders* (Beck and Freeman 1990), which discusses the relations among beliefs, attitudes, and behavior as emanating from cognitive and affective patterns or schemas. For example, Mr. B's paranoid personality disorder (Case 2) would be explained as being associated with a basic belief in his own vulnerability to other people, most of whom he sees as potential adversaries. This results in constant wariness or hypervigilance on his part to guard against the intentions of others. Underdeveloped strategies for the individual with paranoid personality disorder include trust and acceptance. The underlying affect is typically anger or anxiety. Beck and Freeman (1990) provide specific profiles for each of the personality disorders, along with clinical applications for therapy. These could be adapted for the education of patients and their families, leading to more *positive relationships* and patterns of *communication*.

Once the family has been provided with educational information about the patient's personality disorder or style, it may be helpful for the family to provide examples of how the personality traits are expressed and the family's typical response to them. The clinician may observe that problem solving among family members is either ineffective or nonexistent because problems are not dealt with at their source; that is, attitudes and beliefs generate automatic feelings or behaviors.

For many patients and their families, an automatic pattern of *reacting versus responding* contributes to the perpetuation of this situation and is often the result of the family's own frustrations, unmet needs, and feelings, which may vary from guilt and helplessness to rage. The family must be assisted in understanding and containing or managing their own and the patient's uncomfortable feelings in order to defuse difficult or uncomfortable situations and then learn new patterns of responding. This is not unlike the process that most of us learn when we practice controlling our fear and remaining perfectly still while a buzzing bee circles our heads. When this pattern of behavior is repeated over time, the fear of bees becomes bearable or actually disappears as experience leads to the knowledge that the unprovoked insect will eventually fly off without stinging. In psychoanalytic terms, this is known as *accepting the transference,* that is, accepting the projection by the patient onto the therapist of his or her own uncomfortable or negative feelings and attitudes, such as guilt, anger, and helplessness. This is followed by *controlling the countertransference,* or the internal response of the therapist toward the patient, which is at times abetted by the patient's projected affects (Gabbard and Wilkinson 1994).

One model that demonstrates this approach and encourages the family to *accept and set limits* has been developed by Dr. Jerome Kreisman for use with the relatives of individuals with borderline personality disorder. Summarized by the acronym *SET* (support, empathy, truth) (Kreisman and Straus 1989), it consists of three principal components. It is important to emphasize that each component or stage of the SET communication system must be successfully integrated by the patient in order to proceed to the next stage. Likewise, it may be necessary to return to an earlier stage if communication breaks down.

The SET communication system can be illustrated by referring to Case 3 (Mr. C and his mother, who has borderline personality disorder):

1. A statement of *support* that expresses concern, caring, and a desire to be involved with (as opposed to taking care of or responsibility for) the person is the first step in the SET model. For example, as Mr. C prepares to go away with friends for the weekend, his mother calls and asks him to delay going until the next day because she feels a need for his company that evening. When he explains that people are depending on him, she screams at him that he is selfish and does not care about her. He does not react to the anger but rather contains it; nor does he allow it to fuel the guilt he feels each time he goes away. His response, instead, is one of support: "It worries me to know that you're feeling so unhappy right now. I want to help because I love you. I wonder if part of your wanting

me to be around this weekend is because you're missing Joyce" (his mother's vacationing therapist).

When Stage 1 is successfully completed, the patient understands that the speaker is concerned about her.

2. *Empathy*, or the neutral acknowledgment of the other person's feelings, as opposed to sympathy, which may be perceived as devaluation, is the second step in the SET model. To continue the above scenario, Mr. C's mother may respond with tears and a request that Mr. C at least leave later that evening, to which he might say: "I know you're lonely tonight, but we both also know that my staying won't solve the real problem." At this, his mother angrily states that he does not know how she is feeling, and how could he possibly know what her "real" problems are? Mr. C may then agree with her and try another support statement. If successful, he may then attempt to elicit from her a description of her feelings, followed by an attempt to convey his awareness of them: "You have a lot of reasons for feeling that way. It can't be easy for you. I guess we both know that these feelings are something you've struggled with off and on for a long time, and although they aren't just going to go away, I wonder if there are some things you can do to get you through the weekend."

If Mr. C's mother can accept her unpleasant feelings and acknowledge Mr. C's empathy, the next component of the SET model is possible.

3. *Truth* statements are expressed in a neutral way, recognize external factors, and emphasize self-control. If Mr. C successfully proceeds to engage his mother in problem solving her loneliness for the weekend only, he may then explain to her that canceling his own plans at her request would eventually lead to further problems for both of them and would not address long-term issues. He might also reassure her of his continuing support for her by suggesting that they find a mutually convenient time for them to have dinner together when he returns. Truth statements represent reality and emphasize the patient's prime responsibility for her life in a practical, action-oriented manner (*accountability*).

Role-playing examples of typical situations between the family and patient may help to demonstrate the dysfunctional patterns of communicating or reacting and may also allow the practicing of new approaches. The process of *education* and the provision of objective *support* continue throughout these ongoing interactions with the family. It will be helpful for all participants to constantly keep in mind that new and adaptive patterns of coping, behaving, and communicating will be slow for both the patient and the family. The experience of taking positive action, however, especially with the support of an empathic, nonjudgmental clinician, will instill a sense of hope.

In some instances, family members may decide that they can no longer tolerate or accept the patient (or the clinician may suggest this as a potential outcome). In Case 1, for example, Ms. A met with little effort from her husband to work together in order to resolve their difficulties. Individual counseling allowed her to assert and justify her own needs and those of her daughter. At the same time, education provided a more comprehensive understanding of antisocial personality disorder, and she took what she considered to be the healthiest choice for herself and her daughter: divorce.

Throughout the educational and supportive components of working with the family of individuals with personality disorders, it is important to encourage or elicit the family's response to the information provided and strategies suggested (*strengthen communication skills*). This not only facilitates and encourages the interactive approach but also allows opportunities for additional support and empathy, the clarification of perceptions, and the identification of further needs.

Conclusion

The family members of individuals with personality disorders are as much in need of education, information, and support as are any individuals attempting to understand and cope with a baffling, disabling illness. At this early stage in working with these families, the clinician is employing theory-based models and approaches that have been successful with the families of other patient populations. There is reason, however, to have confidence that these models will be appropriate for and beneficial to these families as well as to their members with personality disorders.

Although this model awaits empirical testing, the interventions suggested here will provide the clinician with the necessary background, information, and practical steps in order to proceed.

Suggested Resources

Readings

Beck AT, Freeman A: Cognitive Therapy of Personality Disorders. New York, Guilford, 1990. *Techniques of cognitive therapy that could be used by the clinician and interpreted for use by the family*

Cauwels JM: Imbroglio. New York, Guilford, 1992. *Intended to educate the patient with a diagnosis of borderline personality disorder; extensive coverage but very erudite in terminology and style*

Forward S: Toxic Parents: Overcoming Their Hurtful Legacy. New York, Bantam Books, 1989. *Intended as adjunct to professional therapy in dealing with negative childhood experiences and their impact on current functioning*

Gabbard GO, Wilkinson SM: Management of Countertransference With Borderline Patients. Washington, DC, American Psychiatric Press, 1994. *Extensive definition and use of transference and countertransference techniques for use with patients with severe personality disorders*

Hatfield AB, LeFley HP: Families of the Mentally Ill. New York, Guilford, 1987. *General overview of how family members respond to mental illness and practical ways to assist them*

Kreisman JJ, Straus H: I Hate You—Don't Leave Me: Understanding the Borderline Personality. Los Angeles, CA, The Body Press, Price Stern Sloan, 1989. *Reviews and explains borderline diagnosis, presentation, treatment, and management, including the SET system of communication*

Oldham JM, Morris LB: Personality Self-Portrait: Why You Think, Work, and Act the Way You Do. New York, Bantam Books, 1990. *Good introduction to personality style and disorder, with techniques for interacting with individuals with these disorders; readily understandable*

Organizations

Schizophrenia Society of Canada
Head Office: 75 The Donway West, Suite 815
Don Mills, Ontario, Canada M3C2E9
For all provinces, the local chapter is listed in the telephone directory (except Ontario, which goes under the name Friends of Schizophrenia Society). Offers support and education for families of individuals with disorders whose symptoms and presentation are similar to those of schizophrenia, such as schizoid, schizotypal, and paranoid personality disorders.

Recovery Inc.
Headquarters: 802 North Dearborn Street
Chicago, IL 60610
(In Canada, check white pages of local telephone directory in larger centers.) A North American self-help group with local chapters listed in the telephone directory of most cities. Offers support and an aftercare method for combating nervous ailments. Appropriate for those individuals with personality disorders in which anxiety is a major problem, such as avoidant and obsessive-compulsive personality disorders.

Miscellaneous: Support groups such as Alcoholic Anonymous or Narcotics Anonymous and Manic-Depressive Family Support Groups are potential resources in cases in which another psychiatric disorder coexists with personality disorder. For suggestions on other resources in the United States, contact the National Alliance for the Mentally Ill, Arlington, VA; in Canada, contact the local chapter of the Canadian Mental Health Foundation.

References

Adler G: Uses and limitations of Kohut's self psychology in the treatment of borderline patients. J Am Psychoanal Assoc 37:761–785, 1989

Alden L: Short-term structured treatment for avoidant personality disorder. J Consult Clin Psychol 57:756–764, 1989

American Psychiatric Association: Diagnostic and Statistical Manual of Mental Disorders, 3rd Edition. Washington, DC, American Psychiatric Association, 1980

American Psychiatric Association: Diagnostic and Statistical Manual of Mental Disorders, 4th Edition. Washington, DC, American Psychiatric Association, 1994

Beck AT, Freeman A: Cognitive Therapy of Personality Disorders. New York, Guilford, 1990

Bell NW, Vogel EF: A Modern Introduction to the Family, Revised Edition. New York, Free Press, 1968

Berkowitz R, Eberlein-Fries R, Kuipers L, et al: Educating relatives about schizophrenia. Schizophr Bull 10:418–429, 1984

Brown GW, Birley JLT, Wing JK: Influence of family life on the course of schizophrenic disorders: a replication. Br J Psychiatry 121:241–258, 1972

Cauwels JM: Imbroglio. New York, WW Norton, 1992

Chernen L, Friedman M: Treating the personality disordered agoraphobic patient with individual and marital therapy: a multiple replication study. Journal of Anxiety Disorders 7:163–177, 1993

Deltito JA, Perugi G: A case of social phobia with avoidant personality disorder treated with MAOI. Compr Psychiatry 27:255–258, 1986

Deltito JA, Stam M: Psychopharmacological treatment of avoidant personality disorder. Compr Psychiatry 30:498–504, 1989

DuBrul T: Separation-individuation roller coaster in the therapy of a borderline patient. Perspect Psychiatr Care 25:10–14, 1989

Gabbard GO, Wilkinson SM: Management of Countertransference With Borderline Patients. Washington, DC, American Psychiatric Press, 1994

Goulet J: Passive-aggressive personality and dependent personality: current state of the question. Can J Psychiatry 33:140–146, 1988

Hartman D, Boerger MJ: Families of borderline clients: opening the door to therapeutic interaction. Perspect Psychiatr Care 25:15–17, 1989

Hatfield AB, LeFley HP: Families of the Mentally Ill. New York, Guilford, 1987

Heimberg RG, Barlow DH: New developments in cognitive-behavioral therapy for social phobia. J Clin Psychiatry 52 (suppl):21–30, 1991

Jones SA: Family therapy with borderline and narcissistic patients. Bull Menninger Clin 51:285–295, 1987

Kaplan CA: The challenge of working with patients diagnosed as having a borderline personality disorder. Nurs Clin North Am 21:429–438, 1986

Kreisman JJ, Straus H: I Hate You—Don't Leave Me. Los Angeles, CA, The Body Press, Price Stern Sloan, 1989

Lachkar J: Narcissistic borderline couples: implications for mediation. Conciliation Court Review 24:31–38, 1986

LeFley HP: Culture and mental illness, in Families of the Mentally Ill. Edited by Hatfield AB, LeFley HP. New York, Guilford, 1987, pp 30–59

Mannion MFT, Mueser K, Solomon P: Designing psychoeducational services for spouses of persons with serious mental illness. Community Ment Health J 30:177–190, 1994

Masterson JF: Psychotherapy of borderline and narcissistic disorders: establishing a therapeutic alliance. Journal of Personality Disorders 4:182–191, 1990

Mattick RP, Newman CR: Social phobia and avoidant personality disorder. International Review of Psychiatry 3:163–173, 1991

Maurin JT, Boyd CB: Burden of mental illness on the family: a critical review. Arch Psychiatr Nurs 4:99–107, 1990

McCann JT: Passive-aggressive personality disorder: a review. Journal of Personality Disorders 2:170–179, 1988

Melges FT, Swartz MS: Oscillations of attachment in borderline personality disorder. Am J Psychiatry 146:1115–1120, 1989

Messer AA: Narcissistic people. Medical Aspects of Human Sexuality 19:169–184, 1985

Miller F, Dworkin J, Ward M, et al: A preliminary study of unresolved grief in families of seriously mentally ill patients. Hosp Community Psychiatry 41:1321–1325, 1990

Mitton JM, Links PS, Patrick J, et al: Assessing needs and expressed emotion in the families of borderline personality disordered patients. Poster presented on Annual Poster Day, McMaster School of Nursing, McMaster University, Hamilton, Ontario, Canada, June 1993

Oldham JM: Brief treatment of narcissistic personality disorder. Journal of Personality Disorders 2:88–90, 1988

Oldham JM, Morris LB: Personality Self-Portrait: Why You Think, Work and Act the Way You Do. New York, Bantam Books, 1990

Piccinino S: The nursing care challenge: borderline patients. J Psychosoc Nurs Ment Health Serv 28:23–27, 1990

Renneberg B, Goldstein AJ, Phillips D, et al: Intensive behavioral group treatment of avoidant personality disorder. Behavior Therapy 21:363–377, 1990

Royal Australian and New Zealand College of Psychiatrists: Quality assurance project: treatment outlines for borderline, narcissistic and histrionic personality disorders. Aust N Z J Psychiatry 25:392–403, 1991

Ryglewicz H: Psychoeducation for clients and families: a way in, out and through in working with people with dual disorders. Psychosocial Rehabilitation Journal 15:79–89, 1991

Schulz PM, Schulz SC, Hamer R, et al: The impact of borderline and schizotypal personality disorders on patients and their families. Hosp Community Psychiatry 36:879–881, 1985

Schulz SC, Schulz PM, Wilson WH: Medication treatment of schizotypal personality disorder. Journal of Personality Disorders 2:1–13, 1988

Slavik S, Carlson J, Sperry L: Adlerian marital therapy with the passive-aggressive partner. American Journal of Family Therapy 20:25–35, 1992

Spaniol L, Zipple AM, Lockwood D: The role of the family in psychiatric rehabilitation. Schizophr Bull 18:341–347, 1992

Tonge WL, James DS, Hillam SM: Families without hope: a controlled study of 33 problem families. Br J Psychiatry Special Publication No 11, Royal College of Psychiatrists, 1975

Waldinger RJ: Psychiatry for Medical Students. Washington, DC, American Psychiatric Press, 1984

Wells MC, Glickauf-Hughes C, Buzzell V: Treating obsessive-compulsive personalities in psychodynamic/interpersonal group therapy. Psychotherapy 27:366–379, 1990

Wrate R, Bishop D, Will D: Disability in the Family (videotape). Dundee, Scotland, MACMED, 1987

Index

*Page numbers printed in **boldface** type refer to tables or figures.*